John Lowe

# Medical missions

Their place and power

John Lowe

**Medical missions**
*Their place and power*

ISBN/EAN: 9783741169144

Manufactured in Europe, USA, Canada, Australia, Japa

Cover: Foto ©Andreas Hilbeck / pixelio.de

Manufactured and distributed by brebook publishing software
(www.brebook.com)

John Lowe

**Medical missions**

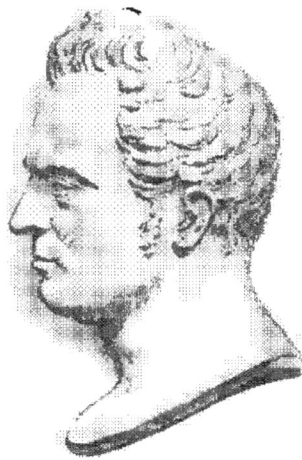

# MEDICAL MISSIONS

## *THEIR PLACE AND POWER.*

BY

## JOHN LOWE, F.R.C.S.E.

SECRETARY OF THE
EDINBURGH MEDICAL MISSIONARY SOCIETY
AND SUPERINTENDENT OF ITS TRAINING INSTITUTION

*WITH INTRODUCTION BY*

## SIR WILLIAM MUIR, K.C.S.I., LL.D., D.C.L.

LATE LIEUTENANT-GOVERNOR NORTH WEST PROVINCES OF INDIA,
AND PRINCIPAL OF THE UNIVERSITY OF EDINBURGH.

London
T FISHER UNWIN
26 PATERNOSTER SQUARE
1886

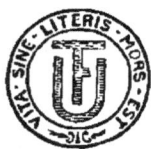
VITA · SINE · LITERIS · MORS · EST · SIC ·

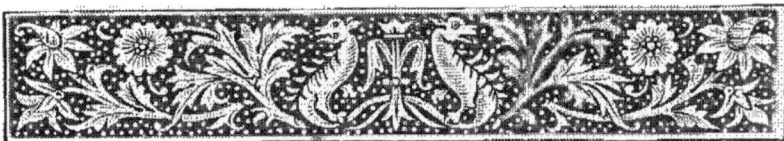

# INTRODUCTION.

I HAVE been asked to write a few lines by way of preface to this volume. I readily do so because fully persuaded of the high value of Medical Missions as an auxiliary to Christian enterprise, and especially in its earliest stage.

The book contains an exhaustive account of the benefits that may, and in point of fact do, accrue from the use of the medical art as a Christian agency. Mr. Lowe is eminently qualified to instruct us in this matter, having himself been so long engaged in the same field. Some, indeed, may be inclined to question whether medical work may not have been too strongly insisted upon here, as a *necessary* branch of all Missionary and Evangelistic agencies ; and it is quite possible, that in enthusiasm for a grand work which has engaged the labour of his life, this view may have been pressed somewhat far. But, however this may be, if we regard medical agencies as the pioneers of regular missions, our Author has not said one word too much in praise of them. In so far as these are used in the breaking of ground yet strange to the Gospel, or amidst needy and outcast classes anywhere, there can hardly be a question in any Christian mind as to their great value. Mr. Lowe has well illustrated this in the instances he has given of the benefits of the healing art

in abating suspicion and prejudice, disarming hostility,
and bespeaking the confidence of the people toward our
Missionaries.    Such, for example, in the experience
gained from the wonderful mission of Dr. Elmslie in
Cashmere, and the practice of the art by well-qualified
Lady physicians in the Harems and Zenanas of the
East.  Throughout Eastern lands, indeed, and especially
amongst Mahometans, the Christian *Hakeem* is always
respected, and always welcome ; and the Gospel which
he carries in one hand is graciously received, because of
the material benefits held out by the other.    And so it
comes to pass, that healing remedies, and kindly treatment of the suffering, become an important means of
making the Missionary popular, and preparing the soil
for reception of the Gospel.

It is, therefore, with high satisfaction, that we learn
from Mr. Lowe of an increasing staff of Medical Missionaries springing up—men able and willing to unite the
office of physician with that of the Christian minister.
And herein, truly, it may be said, that they are but
following the example of our Saviour, who Himself, and
through His disciples, healed the sick simultaneously
with the blessed proclamation that the kingdom of
heaven was at hand.   It is true that miraculous agency
has passed away, but the same analogy still subsists
between the ailments of the body and the soul, and the
disposition is still the same, as of old, in those who are
healed, to listen to the voice of the physician as a preacher
of salvation.   On every ground, therefore, these Medical
Missions are worthy the support of all who have at heart
the success of Missions amongst the poor and in Foreign
lands.                                           W. M.

*March* 11, 1886.

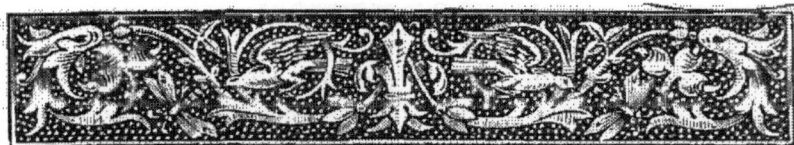

# CONTENTS.

---

### CHAPTER I.

### *THE DIVINE METHOD.*

### CHAPTER II.

### *SPHERE AND SCOPE.*

### CHAPTER III.

### *PIONEER AGENCY.*

## FRONTISPIECE,

# THE DIVINE IDEAL OF "PREACHING THE GOSPEL."

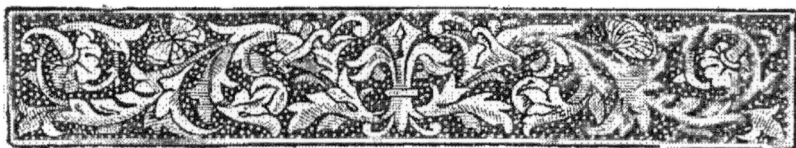

# CHAPTER I.

## The Divine ideal of "Preaching the Gospel" interpreted by our Lord's Ministry and that of His Apostles.

THE missionary enterprise, including the various methods employed in commending God's message of redeeming love to man, is the highest form of Christian benevolence, and the noblest work in which man can engage.

The missionary's theme—the glorious Gospel of the blessed God—is the one only antidote to all the world's sins and sorrows. Its Divine message remains ever the same, "God so loved the world that He gave His only begotten Son, that whosoever believeth in Him should not perish, but have everlasting life," and no circumstance of clime or culture, neither degradation, ignorance, nor prejudice, can weaken its efficacy, or affect its adaptation to the needs of mankind: " For the Gospel is the power of God unto salvation to every one that believeth, to the Jew first, and also to the Greek," and to make known this Gospel is the one aim and object of the missionary enterprise.

The Divine commission, " Go ye into all the world and preach the Gospel to every creature," is, however, much more comprehensive in its meaning, than many of even the most intelligent friends of missions, seem inclined to admit.   The late lamented pioneer of African evangelization, Dr. Livingstone, says truly that " preaching the Gospel to the heathen includes much more than is implied in the usual picture of a missionary—a man going about with a Bible under his arm," indicating, thereby, the grand intention of its Divine Founder, that the Gospel should be proclaimed to mankind not as a mere dogma, but as a life ; that the missionary, while he should maintain a form of sound words, must strive at the same time to commend the Gospel by a practical manifestation of its spirit, and should show to all that, in its beneficent design, it has regard not only to the life that now is, but also to that which is to come.   " How beautiful upon the mountains are the feet of him that bringeth good tidings, that publisheth peace ; " like the fair goddess of whom we read, that, wherever she went, flowers sprang up in her path, so wherever the glorious Gospel of the blessed God is preached in its Divine comprehensiveness, alike by living voice and by loving deeds, there "the wilderness and the solitary place shall be glad, and the desert rejoice and blossom as the rose."

A minister, while visiting in his parish in one of the most destitute and degraded districts of a great city, after ascending a long, dark, winding stair, opened a door leading into a cheerless garret room. There on a pallet of straw, with no covering save her dirty, tattered garments, lay an aged woman, to all appearance dying. Forgetting, for the moment, her outward circumstances, in his anxiety for the welfare of her soul, he inquired with all earnestness whether she had any hope for the world to come. "Oh, sir," she said, as she stretched out her naked, withered arm, "if you were as cold and hungry as I am, you could think of nothing else." That servant of God was taught the lesson that, to succeed in the highest aim of Christian love, our ministry must contemplate man in the whole extent of his being; that the disciple of Christ, in so far as he imbibes the Master's spirit, will walk in the steps of His holy and comprehensive benevolence.

The Lovedale Mission of South Africa, in connection with the Free Church of Scotland, with its college, industrial department, medical mission, and flourishing native churches, is a model which the friends of missions would do well to study. We believe that the directors and supporters of our missionary societies at home, rather than the agents abroad, need to be taught that the great work of evangelizing the heathen ought not to be restricted to any one method, but that every mode of operation that manifests the spirit of the Gospel—every civilizing influence that the missionary can bring to bear upon the people, and that gives to Christianity a practical aspect—every such form of missionary effort, when made to subserve the one great purpose, lies within the scope of the Divine commission, and should have its place in the missionary enterprise.

"If I were asked to explain the success of Lovedale," writes the able Superintendent of that mission, the Rev. Dr. Stewart, "I would say that, under God's blessing, it is chiefly due to the fact that *we proceed on practical lines,* which are always more difficult and laborious, but also more permanent in their effects, than those that are not so ; that the method recognizes man as having a body, as well as a soul ; that while it gives due place and fullest prominence to the life to come, it also recognizes the life that now is, and proceeds on the belief that the future life can be duly, and best, prepared for, by the right performance of the duties of the life we have now. . . . The first preachers were sent to say that the Kingdom of God had come near ; but in support and commendation of that statement, they were also commanded, as well as empowered, to do much of a lower kind of good. These subsidiary efforts, which they were commanded and empowered to put forth, were practical and tangible in their results, appreciable by the senses,

and suited to the material or bodily necessities of those
who were addressed. The directions in the tenth chapter of St. Matthew's Gospel are very explicit, and it is
possible that when first given they were even more
detailed."

And again, Dr. Stewart says : " If it were possible
that to-morrow the Christian benevolence of Great
Britain, or even of London, in all its varied practical
forms, were to be suddenly compelled to assume only
one form—that of preaching—what would become of
the ignorant, the sick, the hungry, and the helpless, of
all sorts and conditions, who are now benefiting by their
benevolence, taking on a multitude of shapes in addition
to the one which stimulates and perfects them all, and
which gives them a value beyond the present time ?
Would the Christian Church itself be benefited by such
a change ? Or would the experience that has been
gained as to what is necessary to be done, if we would
reach the hearts of the helpless and despairing, in order
to rouse them from the stupor of their misery and gain
their ear, either endorse or accept that view ? The
heathen abroad, in uncivilized countries at least, correspond to the morally helpless and despairing at home ; all
the more closely do they correspond in those countries
that lie adjacent to, or form part of, the territories of
civilization, where their struggle for existence, and con-
tinuance on their own soil, is severely felt ; and where
that civilization comes sweeping in upon them with great

power, for evil as well as for good, and finds them unable
to resist the one, or ready to accept the other, without
guidance or assistance.   This assistance, within certain
limits, in its earliest stages, must be given by the missionary, if it is to be given at all—just as at home, the
corresponding work is to be mainly done by the Christian Church, or left undone."

We, at home, can hardly realize the difficulties that
a missionary has to contend with in his efforts to introduce the Gospel into heathen, and often uncivilized,
countries.   Here, we are surrounded with every Christian
influence, and with benevolent institutions and organiza-
tions which testify, more emphatically than words, to the
enlightening, humanizing, regenerating power of Christianity.   We have our colleges and schools, our hospitals
for the sick, asylums for the insane and for the blind,
refuges for the destitute, homes for the fallen and outcast, associations for the relief of the aged and for
improving the condition of the poor, reformatories for
wayward and neglected children, and agencies without
number to counteract almost every form of evil, and to
meet every conceivable requirement.   These auxiliaries
to the Church's aggressive work are everywhere in active
operation, and are generously supported, as the practical
outcome of our Christianity, and are deemed essentially
necessary to the successful prosecution of home missionary work.   The missionary to the heathen, on the other
hand, settles down among a people ignorant, super-

stitious, and degraded, it may be, where no humanizing influences are at work, but where, on the contrary, the strong oppress the weak—where the sick are uncared for, or treated with barbarous cruelty—where the aged and infirm are counted a burden, and either perish from neglect or linger on in misery—where the arts and usages of civilization are unknown—where, in short, little or no vestige of anything but sin is to be seen. Under circumstances such as these, what can the missionary do? "Preach the Gospel," we say, for the "glorious Gospel of our blessed God" is the one only panacea for all the world's miseries. Yes, the Gospel is the "power of God" —the power which has made Britain a land of greatness, intelligence, and influence, beyond any other nation on the face of the globe ; it is the power which, again and again, has broken the arm of oppression and tyranny, and, dispelling from the minds of millions the dark clouds of ignorance and superstition, has raised the beggar from the dung-hill and set him among princes ; it is the power which, having tamed and humanized the savage nature, has chased idolatry from many a heathen land and from many of the islands of the sea, and which shall yet, everywhere, cause the "wilderness to be like Eden, and the desert like the garden of the Lord." Yes, but much more is implied in "preaching the Gospel" than the mere proclamation of the Divine message. The heathen can best be taught as little children are instructed in our schools—by object lessons. The

Gospel must therefore be preached to them, alike by the living voice, and by the unmistakable evidence of loving deeds.    Like the Apostle Paul, the true missionary, the workman that needeth not to be ashamed, must be able to say, " By word and deed, I have fully preached unto the Gentiles the Gospel of Christ."   The Gospel means " Glad tidings," and preaching the Gospel means the setting forth of the best of all glad tidings—the love of God to man.   To the heathen abroad, as well as to the godless at home, the most convincing proof of the reality and power of that love is, that it begets love for man ; and wherever, in carrying on our evangelistic operations, this practical demonstration of the power of the Gospel is withheld, the Gospel is not "fully preached."   "If a brother or sister be naked, and destitute of daily food, and one of you say unto them, Depart in peace, be ye warmed and filled ; notwithstanding ye give them not those things which are needful for the body, what doth it profit ?   Even so, faith, if it hath not works, is dead, being alone."   " Faith, hope, charity, these three ; but the greatest of these is charity "—love to God, begetting love for man ; and what is the aim and object of Christian love?   It is the welfare of my brother, the welfare of his body, the welfare of his soul—his welfare for time, his welfare for eternity.   To hold forth the Word of Life, along with a practical manifestation of the spirit of the Gospel, is therefore the true meaning of " Preaching the Gospel," and this is the aim and object of Medical Missions, an enterprise which claims alike the sympathy of the Christian and the Philanthropist. We believe that the Divine meaning of "preaching the Gospel" implies something more than the teaching of a dogma, than the mere proclamation of the Gospel message; that, as He who is the sum and substance of the Gospel "was made flesh and dwelt among us"—that, as He sympathized with suffering humanity, fed the hungry, healed the sick, and went about continually doing good, thus manifesting the spirit of His own religion, and teaching, by loving deeds, its principles, so His ambassadors must "preach the Gospel," not by word only, but likewise by a benevolent, Christlike ministry, performed in Christ's name and for His sake.

The evangelization of the world is Christ's own work, and those who, as His instruments, are called to engage in it, are commissioned to represent Christ—to represent Him in all His tender pity for the lost, His loving sympathy with the afflicted, His care for the sick, His compassion for the suffering. We turn therefore to Christ's ministry on earth for the interpretation of His own commission, " Go ye into all the world, and preach the Gospel to every creature."

In reading the New Testament, one cannot fail to be struck with the fact, that our Lord's personal ministry on earth, as well as that of His Apostles, was pre-eminently the work of the medical missionary.

In the last three verses of the fourth chapter of St.

Matthew's Gospel, we read: "And Jesus went about all Galilee, teaching in their synagogues, and preaching the Gospel of the Kingdom, and healing all manner of sickness and all manner of disease among the people; and His fame went throughout all Syria; and they brought unto Him all sick people that were taken with divers diseases and torments, and those that were lunatic, and those that had the palsy, and He healed them; and there followed Him great multitudes of people from Galilee, and from Decapolis, and from Jerusalem, and from Judæa, and from beyond Jordan."

Jesus was just then entering upon His public ministry. He knew man's heart—the way to gain access to it—its prejudices, and the many obstacles in the way of the people receiving His teaching; and, knowing all this, such was the means He employed to reveal His character and claims, to remove prejudice, and to draw men to Himself. By the exercise of His healing power, He gathered round Him a great congregation, with hearts overflowing with gratitude, and thus the searching truths of the "Sermon on the Mount" fell as living seed upon a prepared soil.

Having finished His sermon on the mount, He immediately resumes His ministry of healing, and "when He was come down from the mountain, great multitudes followed Him: and, behold there came a leper and worshipped Him, saying, Lord, if thou wilt, thou canst make me clean. And Jesus put forth His hand and

touched him, saying, I will, be thou clean ; and immediately his leprosy was cleansed." His first act was to
heal a leper ; His second, to cure the centurion's servant,
sick of the palsy and grievously tormented ; His third,
to restore Peter's wife's mother, sick of a fever; and then,
"when the even was come, they brought unto Him many
that were possessed with devils, and He cast out the
spirits with His word, and healed all that were sick."

Following the sacred narrative, down to the close of the
ninth chapter of St. Matthew's Gospel we find it to be just a
record (to use modern phraseology) of Christ's itinerant
medical missionary work, concluding with these words,
"And Jesus went about all the cities and villages, teaching
in their synagogues, and preaching the Gospel of the
Kingdom, and healing every sickness and every disease
among the people."

When we inquire into the character of our Lord's
miracles, we find that no fewer than twenty-three, or two-
thirds of the whole, were miracles of healing, and it is
evident that those which are recorded are but a few,
compared with the many of which no details are given.
When the Pharisees were consulting together how they
might destroy Him, Jesus, we read, "withdrew Himself,
and great multitudes followed Him, and He healed them
all " (Matt. xii. 15). After having cured the daughter of
the woman of Canaan, He departed from the coasts of
Tyre and Sidon "and came nigh unto the sea of Galilee,
and went up into a mountain, and sat down there ; and

great multitudes came unto Him, having with them those
that were lame, blind, dumb, maimed, and many others,
and cast them down at Jesus' feet, and He healed them"
(Matt. xv. 30). Departing from Galilee, "He came into
the coasts of Judæa beyond Jordan, and great multitudes
followed Him, and He healed them there." (Matt. xix.
1, 2). Having returned to Jerusalem, "the blind and
the lame came to Him in the temple, and He healed
them" (Matt. xxi. 14). And again, in (Luke iv. 40), we
read, "Now when the sun was setting, all they that had
any sick with divers diseases brought them unto Him,
and He laid His hands on every one of them and healed
them."

If there is one feature more prominent than another
in the record of our Lord's ministry on earth, it is the
exercise of healing power which, everywhere and on
all occasions, He displayed. These miracles of healing
are not to be regarded as mere proofs of Christ's
divinity; this, they no doubt were, for when John heard
of His mighty works he sent two of His disciples to ask,
"Art thou He that should come, or do we look for
another? Jesus answering, said unto them, Go your
way, and tell John what things ye have seen and heard,
how that the blind see, the lame walk, the lepers are
cleansed, the deaf hear, the dead are raised, to the poor
the Gospel is preached." "My works," He said, "pro-
claim me to be the Son of God, and the promised
Messiah, concerning whom the prophet wrote, 'He hath

anointed me to preach the Gospel to the poor, He hath
sent me to heal the broken-hearted, to preach deliverance to the captives, and recovering of sight to the
blind, to set at liberty them that are bruised, to preach
the acceptable year of the Lord.'" These miraculous
works of healing were unanswerable proofs that He was,
what He claimed to be, the Son of God; but they were
more—they were living manifestations of the spirit of
His own religion, they spoke a language intelligible to
every human conscience: while they declared Him to
be the Son of God with power, they at the same time
revealed His tender compassion, His loving sympathy,
His incomprehensible love, and in this light His own
disciples regarded them as the fulfilment of the words
spoken by Esaias, the prophet, "Himself took our
infirmities and bare our sicknesses." Nor is this manifestation of sympathy with human suffering confined
alone to our Lord's miracles of healing. " Having
compassion on the multitude," is the key that unlocks
the meaning of nearly all His "mighty works;" and in
many of the parables by which He taught the people,
as in His ordinary familiar intercourse with them and
His disciples, the same deep compassion for, and
sympathy with, human suffering are constantly displayed.

As the Divine Author and Founder of Christianity,
the record of our Lord's personal ministry must ever be
to us deeply suggestive and instructive. Every feature
of that ministry claims our devout attention. His mode

of commending the truth, in so far as it was super-
natural, we cannot imitate, but, in so far as it was intended as a manifestation of the spirit of the Gospel (as
much needed now as then), " He hath left us an example
that we should follow in His steps."

This aspect of our Lord's personal ministry brings us
face to face with the Divine idea of preaching the
Gospel—an idea which attaches very special importance
to the method, and strikingly illustrates the principle of
medical missions; so much so, indeed, that the impartial
student of Christ's life must be impressed with the
conviction, that of all the methods employed by the
Church as auxiliaries to her missionary work, this is the
most Christ-like.

We have not only our Lord's example, but also what
is perhaps more emphatic, His direct command ; what He
Himself did, He commissioned His Apostles and the
first teachers of Christianity to do. " And when He
had called unto Him His twelve disciples, He gave
them power against unclean spirits, to cast them out,
and to heal all manner of sickness and all manner of
disease" (Matt. x. 1). "And after these things, the
Lord appointed other seventy also, and sent them, two
and two, before His face into every city and place,
whither He Himself would come" (Luke x. 1). To them
He gave a similar commission, "And into whatsoever
city ye enter, . . . heal the sick that are therein, and say
unto them, The kingdom of God is come nigh unto you "

(Luke x. 8, 9). The manner in which they fulfilled their commission is fully recorded in the inspired account of the history of the primitive Church. What, indeed, is the book of the Acts of the Apostles, but the first report of the first Medical Missionary Society? Therein we find recorded such incidents as: "By the hands of the apostles were many signs and wonders wrought among the people; insomuch that they brought forth the sick into the streets, and laid them on beds and couches, that at least the shadow of Peter passing by might overshadow some of them. There came also a multitude out of the cities round about unto Jerusalem, bringing sick folks, and them which were vexed with unclean spirits; and they were healed every one" (Acts v. 12, 15, 16). Again, we read, "Philip went down to the city of Samaria, and preached Christ unto them. And the people with one accord gave heed unto those things which Philip spake, hearing and seeing the miracles which he did. For unclean spirits, crying with loud voice, came out of many that were possessed with them; and many taken with palsies, and that were lame, were healed; and there was great joy in that city" (Acts viii. 5–8). Scarcely had Paul and Barnabas begun their missionary tour, than we read of Paul healing the impotent man at Lystra, who "had been a cripple from his mother's womb, and never had walked," and by the exercise of healing power so arrested the attention of the people, and drew forth their gratitude, that they

3

brought oxen and garlands, and, thinking that Paul and
Barnabas were "gods come down to them in the likeness
of men," the priests with the people prepared to offer
sacrifice to them, and thus an opportunity was given to
the Apostles of declaring the Gospel to the Gentiles, and
of urging them "to turn from their vanities to serve the
living God" (Acts xiv. 8–18). During our own medical
missionary experience in South India, we have repeatedly
seen this incident almost literally enacted.

Looking to the New Testament, therefore, for guidance as to the methods which ought to be employed by
the Church in her missionary operations, it is, we
think, plainly taught that Christ and His disciples
preached the Gospel "by word and deed," and that the
more we incorporate the healing of the sick with our
evangelistic efforts, the more closely do we follow the
Divine example, and the more fully do we obey the
Master's command.

It may be said, however, that it was by the forth-
putting of His own Divine power that Christ did these
mighty works which spread His fame throughout all
Syria, and that it was in virtue of miraculous endow-
ments (now no longer available) that His disciples made
the deaf to hear, the blind to see, and the lame to walk,
and that therefore their method cannot be intended as
a model for our imitation. Such an inference would be
legitimate, were these miracles of healing intended merely
as attestations to the Divinity of Christ, and as proofs of

the Divine origin of the Gospel: but, as we have already seen, they were more than this—they were a practical manifestation of the compassionate spirit of the Gospel; they spoke, in a language that could not be misunderstood, of Him who came "not to destroy men's lives, but to save them ;" and surely, in so far as this was the object of these "mighty works," they are recorded for our instruction, teaching us that, in our missionary enterprises, the consecration of the healing art to the service of the Gospel is not only in accordance with the Divine method, but actually forms part of the Divine intention.

"And He sent them to preach the kingdom of God, and to heal the sick." "Go ye into all the world, and preach the Gospel to every creature." On two different occasions these twofold commissions were given by our Lord to His disciples, and through them to us. Is the one binding upon the Church now, and the other not? In fulfilment of our Lord's parting commission, the Church has accepted the responsibility, notwithstanding the fact that the "gift of tongues" is not now, as then, miraculously bestowed, but the qualification which it conveyed must be patiently and laboriously acquired. Shall the command of our Lord in reference to "healing the sick," which formed so prominent a feature of His own ministry and that of His Apostles, be ignored, because what He and they did by the exercise of miraculous power can now be accomplished only by the use of means ? We shall find, further on, illustration of the power of this agency in opening up the way for the Missionary of the Cross, and, in view of this, such an argument will have little weight. Nay, rather, the withdrawal of miraculous endowment renders it all the more imperative that we cultivate and consecrate, with the utmost energy and devotion, not only the science of philology, but also that of medicine, that so we may fulfil our Lord's commission in all its breadth and fulness, and, following His example, preach the Gospel "by word and deed."

Apart altogether from such considerations as these, may we not find evidence in the inspired record of ordinary medical skill having its acknowledged place in the Christian system? In the reference made by the Apostle James to anointing the sick with oil, and praying over them, all who are familiar with Eastern manners and customs know that inunction with oil is the most common of all native remedies. Lightfoot, commenting on James v. 14, says, "Anointing with oil was an ordinary medicinal application to the sick. If we take the Apostle's counsel as referring to this medicinal practice, we may construe it, that he would have this physical administration to be improved to the best advantage, namely, that whereas 'anointing with oil' was ordinarily used to the sick by way of physic, he advises that they should send for the Elders of the Church to do it, that they, with the applying of this corporal physic, might also pray with and for the patient, and apply the spiritual physic of good admonition and comfort to him."

Then, again, in the choice of Luke, "the beloved physician," as his travelling companion, may we not infer St. Paul's recognition of the value of the medical element in the evangelist? Luke met Paul at Troas on the Apostle's journey from Galatia to Macedonia. During his visit to Galatia Paul suffered from some form of bodily affliction, and from his allusion to the readiness of the Galatians to show their devotion to him by plucking out their own eyes if it had been possible and giving them to him, it is supposed that his infirmity was some affection of the eyes. From the "thorn in the flesh" he had again and again by prayer sought miraculous deliverance, but received in answer the promise of all-sufficient grace to sustain him in his affliction. St. Paul was taught that miraculous power is not to be exercised to make life less a sacrifice and burden to God's servants. Jesus Himself never used this power to make life easier to Himself; consequently when Paul's trouble was not to be miraculously removed, what more natural than that he should avail himself of the best medical skill he could command? And hence, hearing of Luke's conversion and of his skill as a physician, he seeks the benefit of his advice, and secures his co-operation in the prosecution of his mission; and by and by, when Paul left Luke at Philippi, where he continued to labour for some seven years, may he not be regarded as a medical missionary placed in charge of the infant Philippian Church? Viewing his position in this light, Neander observes : "His skill would be very useful in securing many an opportunity for publishing the Gospel among the heathen. Christianity, in its earliest stages, used miracles to confirm as well as to embody its Divine message of mercy to mankind; but even in Apostolic times we have indications that medical skill and devotedness were employed to open the way for the Gospel messenger." [1]

Thus far have we endeavoured to show that, while the Gospel is the one only antidote to all the world's sins and sorrows, to prove effectual it must be proclaimed by living witnesses to its transforming power, and its Divine energy must be manifested in a living embodiment of its beneficent design—that He Himself " went about continually doing good," and when He sent forth His disciples to evangelize, He said unto them, "Heal the sick, and say unto them, The kingdom of God is come nigh unto you ;" that, indeed, teaching, preaching, and healing the sick are closely interwoven with the entire history of New Testament missionary operations. We have tried to point out, further, that while this ministry of healing was exercised by miraculous interposition, yet there is no reason why the Church should neglect this duty ; because, in so far as these " mighty works " were performed as the outcome

[1] We refer the reader to an interesting and suggestive paper on this subject, entitled " Luke, the Beloved Physician," by the Rev. Robert McCheyne Edgar, M.A., in the *British and Foreign Evangelical Review* for April, 1883.

and embodiment of the spirit of the Gospel, it is in the power of the Church still to manifest the same compassion by the adoption of the very same means—by the consecration of medical science to the service of the Gospel, and, moreover, there is evidence in the sacred narrative that such is the Divine intention.

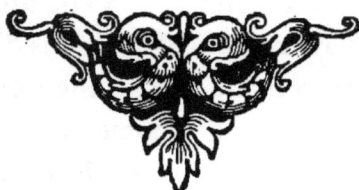

# THE SPHERE AND SCOPE OF MEDICAL MISSIONS.

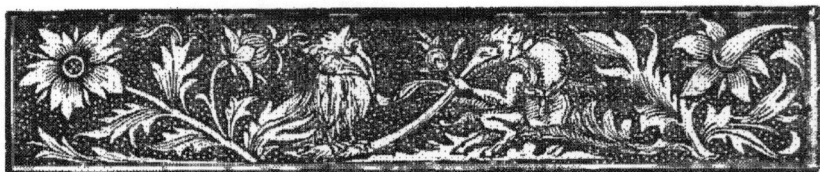

## CHAPTER II.

**The sphere and scope of Medical Missions, and the Medical Missionary's qualifications, status, and method of work.**

IT might have been expected that the facts referred to, regarding our Lord's personal ministry and that of His Apostles, and which stand out so prominently in the New Testament narrative, would have naturally suggested to the fathers and founders of the modern missionary enterprise the idea of incorporating medical missions with their earliest efforts. Strange to say, however, medical missions are yet in their infancy, and although, wherever established, their value has been abundantly proved, and although the needs of the heathen, as well as of the missionaries and their families, are so manifest, yet, even in this age of practical evangelistic activity, their very existence is known to comparatively few, and too many of

these, we fear, have but a vague idea of what a medical
mission really is.   Such misconceptions regarding the
aims and objects of medical missions exist even in our
Mission Boards, that recently, in answer to the application
of a most promising medical missionary student for an
appointment, the following official reply was given :—
" It is not our province to send out and support medical
men in charge of dispensaries and hospitals in our mission
fields.   Our agents are sent forth to preach the Gospel to
the heathen."   Such a reply indicates not only a want of
sympathy with the work, but a complete misconception
as to the nature and objects of medical missions.   It is
essentially necessary, therefore, that the position and
functions of the medical missionary should be clearly
understood before the claims of his work can be duly
appreciated, and these we shall proceed, as briefly as
possible, to define.

From a merely humanitarian point of view, and as a
purely philanthropic agency, our missionary societies are
not called upon to send forth, nor would they be justified in supporting physicians, as such, in charge of
hospitals and dispensaries in connection with their
missions.   It is for the *evangelization* of the heathen that
our missionary societies exist ; for this purpose their
resources are provided, and for this object only can they
be legitimately applied.   The sacred, solemn trust committed to the Directorate of these societies, is to discover
and employ such agencies only as bear the stamp of the

Divine approval, embody the spirit of the Gospel, and shall most effectually accomplish the object in view. Various evangelistic methods have been employed as auxiliary agencies in connection with the missionary enterprise, and it is as one of these that we advocate medical missions.

The function, *par excellence*, of the medical missionary is that of the evangelist. He claims to be as truly a missionary, in the ecclesiastical sense of the word, as his ministerial brother ; both have been educated and trained for the same great work, and both are equally unworthy of the name they bear if they fail to make evangelistic work the grand aim and object of their presence in the mission field. We emphasize this view of the medical missionary's sphere and function; first, and foremost, must be his missionary qualifications, and from a missionary standpoint the success of his work must be estimated. This is no theoretical view of the medical missionary's position. No *true* missionary physician would be satisfied with any other, and no missionary society would be justified in sending forth to engage in this ministry a missionary physician whose estimate of his work is lower.

Let us not, however, be misunderstood. While maintaining that the true position and function of the medical missionary is that of the evangelist, we by no means under-estimate the importance of his strictly professional qualifications. In this, as in all other departments of missionary service, the consecration of the very highest attainments is not only desirable, but necessary. Indeed, none but men whose professional abilities are above the average should be accepted for this department of service. The circumstances in which the missionary physician may be placed, are much more exacting, and necessitate a far greater amount of professional skill and self-reliance, than is the case in this country. Here, when complications and difficulties are met with in practice, the physican may obtain the help of a brother practitioner, who will share with him the responsibility—while there, as a rule, the medical missionary finds himself located where no such help can be obtained. On the contrary, till he shall have trained from among the natives his own assistants, he must act as dispenser, dresser, and nurse; he must be his own consulting physician and surgeon, and himself be president, committee, and officer of the Local Board of Health, architect, master-builder, medical staff, purveyor, and general superintendent of his hospital and dispensary. He must be qualified to teach to others the principles and practice of his profession ; he must be prepared for, all emergencies, not in one, but in all departments of his professional work. Probably he will not be long in the field, before he will be called upon to treat cases which will tax his skill and self-reliance to the utmost; and these, it must be borne in mind, are the very cases which, from a medical missionary point of view, make their influence felt, either for or against the one great object in view—the opening of the door for the proclamation of the Gospel message. It is not the cases that require little or no skill in their treatment— not cases which the *Hakim* or native physician can somehow cure as successfully, perhaps, as the European doctor; but the cases which will pioneer the way for the missionary, and open the fountain of gratitude, and, with God's blessing, prepare the heart to receive God's message of redeeming love, are just such as the skilled hand only can relieve, and the accomplished and thoroughly trained physician alone can understand and treat. For this department of service, therefore, no ordinary professional qualifications will do; the work demands, and surely it may claim, the consecration of the best talents and the highest accomplishments.

We cannot help here deprecating, very strongly, the plan adopted by some missionary societies of giving their students a very partial training in medicine and surgery, and sending them forth as medical missionaries. In no department of service is it more true than in the practice of medicine, that "a little knowledge is a dangerous thing." It is no light responsibility to under- take the treatment of disease, especially in circumstances such as these in which the missionary is so often placed; and yet, for such a responsible duty, some of our mission boards are satisfied with men, whose knowledge of the healing art is just sufficient to reveal their utter incapacity when their help is called for in cases of serious illness, severe accidents, or other emergencies. The Directors

of our missionary societies would, we doubt not, be
among the first to protest against such a reprehensible
system in providing for the medical relief of our poor at
home, or even of the convicts in our gaols. For the
medical care of our native troops in India and elsewhere,
none but the very best men are selected, and, moreover,
they must undergo a prolonged and special course of
instruction in tropical diseases before they are placed in
charge. Shall.only duly qualified and competent men be
eligible for the service of our Queen and country, and
men who have acquired only a very limited knowledge of
medicine, and no legal qualifications, be deemed suffi-
ciently qualified for the service of Christ in the mission
field? Surely there is something wrong if such a principle has the sanction and approval of the Church! If
it were the case that fully qualified men, constrained by
the love of Christ, are not available to meet the requirements of the missionary enterprise—while it would be
humiliating for the Church of Christ to have to make
such a confession, and dishonouring to the noble profession of medicine, from the ranks of which there is no
lack of candidates for all other services—there would,
in such circumstances, be some excuse for our missionary
societies accepting partially educated men for this department of work; but there are, at this moment, not a
few medical men in practice, in cities and towns throughout our land, and many young medical students at our
Universities and medical schools, burning with the

desire to consecrate their life, energies, and talents, upon the missionary altar—waiting for the Church's call, and ready to respond to it. Let the Church awake to her duty and responsibility in regard to this enterprise, and let our missionary societies cordially invite the co-operation of medical missionaries, and we do not hesitate to assert that there will be no lack of earnest, devoted, enthusiastic candidates, for this Christ-like service in the high places of the field.

We do not object to a missionary student acquiring what knowledge of medicine he can, before going forth to his work. In all ordinary cases of illness, in his own family, and among the people, such knowledge will prove of service, but we protest against such partially trained men being sent out by our missionary societies as guardians of the health of their missionaries, and as their accredited agents to treat the diseases of the people, so long as thoroughly educated and fully qualified medical missionaries are prepared, at the call of the Church, to say, "Here am I, send me."

Let it then be clearly understood, that when we speak of medical missionaries we do not mean missionaries with a partial knowledge of medicine, acquired, somehow, while prosecuting their theological studies; but we mean men who, having given good evidence that they possess evangelistic gifts, and the true missionary spirit, have systematically studied medicine and surgery, and have obtained legal qualifications to practise.

A question of great practical importance here suggests itself. The medical missionary goes forth to the mission field as an evangelist. His primary object is identical with that of his clerical colleague. Should not the medical missionary, therefore, be formally "set apart" to the work, and his missionary character and claims be officially recognized by the Church? We venture to say, that our missionary societies are making a mistake in sending forth their medical missionaries without, in some way, solemnly and publicly recognizing them as " the messengers of the churches." We believe this omission accounts for much of the misapprehension, so prevalent, regarding the nature of the medical missionary's work, and the position he ought to occupy in the mission field ; even in his own estimation, his sphere and function are apt to assume a less spiritual aspect than they otherwise would, and the temptation to withdraw from direct missionary work, and to cultivate private practice, is consequently less easily resisted. We can testify from experience, that the fact of having been solemnly "set apart " to the work of the Lord, fortifies the medical missionary, in no small degree, to withstand such allurements.

The question next arises, as to the form which the ecclesiastical recognition of the medical missionary should assume—to what office shall he be "set apart?" We have had intimations sent to us from some of our great missionary societies, that they can accept as medical

missionaries such only as are prepared to offer themselves
for ordination to the office of the ministry.  That is to
say, that fully qualified young men, inspired with the
true missionary spirit, offering themselves for this service,
instead of being sent forth at once to their work, shall
forego medical practice for two, three, or four years, as
the case may be, and devote themselves to theological
study, in order that they may be eligible for ordination.
Now, nothing is more important for a medical student,
on obtaining his degree, than that he should immediately
avail himself of opportunities for gaining practical professional experience.  Any prolonged delay in applying
the knowledge he has acquired will assuredly prove
prejudicial to his future professional success.  We hold,
therefore, that it is unreasonable to expect that a young
man, at the close of his medical curriculum, should,
for a longer or shorter period, abandon professional
work, in order to engage in a course of theological study,
just at the time when he should be turning his theoretical
knowledge to practical account.  Is it, however, really
desirable that the medical missionary should receive
ordination to the office of the ministry?  Most emphatically and without hesitation, we say that, as a rule, it is
not.  In view of the position which we claim for him,
does it not seem unreasonable to expect, that while the
missionary physician is enthusiastically engaged in his
own special sphere, he should at the same time be
required to undertake the duties of the clerical mis-

sionary? We know of several instances where, owing to the want of a due appreciation of this agency on the part of home committees, most accomplished missionary physicians have been sent out as ordained clerical agents, and have had, like other missionaries, pastoral and educational work assigned to them, and, consequently, their usefulness and influence as medical missionaries have been scarcely appreciable.

We plead with all earnestness that our medical missionaries be ordained or "set apart " to their work; but their work, we maintain, is not that of the pastor— not that of presiding over and organizing native churches and mission schools, and superintending the native evangelists and teachers. The medical missionary will, as he has time and opportunity, co-operate with his clerical colleague in all such work, but the proper calling of the medical missionary is that of the evangelist, and to the office and work of the evangelist, therefore, let him be "set apart." Let him, after due examination as to his evangelistic qualifications, be officially recognized and sent forth, with the *imprimatur* of the Church to which he belongs, as her duly accredited messenger to the heathen; and, further, let such recognition imply that, in the exceptional circumstances in which he may sometimes be placed, with no ministerial brother at hand, he may when required dispense the ordinances of the Church. Surely no section of the Church of Christ is so fettered by conventional forms, that she will refuse to

confer such a recognition upon those whom she sends
forth as her representatives to the heathen to engage in
this Christ-like work.

To our mind, there is certainly much more scriptural
authority for " setting apart " the medical missionary as
an evangelist, than there is for ordaining to the office of
the ministry the missionary sent forth to superintend
educational work, whose time and strength must necessarily, and to a very large extent, be devoted to secular
teaching.   The Great Head of the Church, we are told,
called His twelve disciples together, " and He sent them
two and two before His face into every city and place,
and said unto them, Heal the sick that are therein, and
say unto them, The kingdom of God is come nigh unto
you."   We are taught, moreover, that the evangelist is as
much a Divine gift to the Church as is the pastor.   " He
gave some apostles, and some prophets; and some
evangelists, and some pastors and teachers, for the per-
fecting of the saints, for the work of the ministry, for the
edifying of the body of Christ."

What we ask the Church to do, therefore, is just what
the Great Head of the Church Himself did—to recognize the medical missionary as an evangelist, one of
God's appointed gifts, and to send him forth to his
work as much the accredited ambassador of the Church
as his ministerial colleague.

A few years ago the following memorial on this subject
was addressed by the " Edinburgh Medical Missionary

Society" to the Foreign Mission Committee of the Free Church of Scotland, and to the Mission Boards of the other Churches in the United Kingdom :—

"The Directors desire to memorialize the Committee on Foreign Missions in regard to a subject which is growing rapidly in importance, and seems to claim the attention of all evangelical churches. It is the *ecclesiastical status* of the medical missionary. They take this step in the hope and expectation that the Committee on Foreign Missions will aid them in bringing the subject before the General Assembly, for the sake of those students of the Livingstone Memorial Training Institution who happen to be engaged as agents in their service, or are members of their communion. In doing so, it seems proper to mention that they contemplate the transmission of a similar memorial to the Foreign Mission Boards of the other churches in Scotland, England, and Ireland.

"The following considerations, stated as concisely as possible, will indicate the line of thought which has led them to conclude that every medical missionary ought to receive ecclesiastical recognition.

"1. It is an obvious duty of the Christian Church to sympathize with, and encourage, every scriptural method of carrying out the Master's farewell injunction.

"2. The medical mission principle is in close accordance with the example both of the Lord Himself, and of His immediate followers, and experience amply attests the value of this form of mission agency.

"3. Hitherto, the medical missionary, however competent, both as a thoroughly-educated professional man, and as a trained evangelist, has never received any ecclesiastical recognition, unless, in addition to his professional qualifications, he has passed through a more or less complete curriculum of theological study, entitling him, after due presbyterial examination, to receive license as a probationer.

"4. A few exceptional instances, it is true, have been met with, in which this combination has proved satisfactory, but to regard it as *essential* would prove a serious impediment to the cause of medical missions. The study of surgery and medicine now covers so wide a field, that it taxes the mental energies of students—of those especially who aim at exceptional eminence—so that, to do any justice to a complete theological course, pursued simultaneously, would be simply impossible; while for a young medical man to address himself to the latter, after he had acquired his diploma or degree, would be very prejudicial to his prospects of future usefulness in his profession. A course of theology, extending over three or four years, would have the inevitable effect of preventing him from acquiring that practical experience which is so essential, and of blunting the edge of all his previous attainments. The result would certainly be to mar him as a surgeon.

"5. No young man is admitted as a student of the Livingstone Memorial Institution until his personal re-

ligious history, his missionary spirit, and his general
qualifications for missionary work have been carefully
inquired into ; his medical studies are thereafter pursued
at the Edinburgh School of Medicine—either intra-mural
or extra-mural—and all the time (four years) while
breathing, so to speak, a mission atmosphere, he becomes practically familiar with evangelistic work, in its
various aspects.    What the Directors desire is this : that
having got the *imprimatur* of the Medical School as a
surgeon and physician, he should also get the *imprimatur*
of the Church before going forth to the foreign field as a
medical missionary.

"The Directors would suggest that, after a reasonable,
tender, considerate examination by a Presbyterial Committee, he should be set apart, or ordained, as an evangelist—a designation not new to the Presbyterian churches,
applicable also, as we imagine, to the case of churches
other than Presbyterian, and, moreover, a designation
accurately descriptive of his rightful office and work.

"In thoroughly-equipped missions, the medical missionary might occupy the position of ruling elder, so as
to strengthen the hands of the clerical missionary, and
aid him in forming a session ; but in pioneer missions—
for which the medical missionary seems specially suited—
his *status* as evangelist, for which the Directors are now
pleading, might reasonably admit of his dispensing seal-
ing ordinances, when these happen to be called for in
exceptional circumstances.    Of course, should an or-

dained clerical missionary be eventually added to the mission, the medical evangelist would retire, for the time at least, from the performance of these functions."

This memorial was very favourably received by the Mission Boards of the various churches, and the assurance was given that its proposals would be carefully considered by their Directors, while the Foreign Mission Committee of the Free Church of Scotland, and the Mission Board of the United Presbyterian Church, have already, to a great extent, adopted the suggestions, and, before sending them forth to the mission field, their medical missionaries are now formally and publicly recognised as the Church's ambassadors to the heathen.

With regard to the training of the medical missionary, enough has been said to show that his professional education must be thorough and comprehensive ; and, it should be added, specially so in surgery. Natives, almost everywhere, have a kind of intuitive knowledge of the medicinal virtue of indigenous plants, and although they are, as a rule, utterly ignorant of the diseases they presume to treat, yet much confidence is placed in the native doctors and their nostrums, and, somehow, they do at times appear to effect wonderful cures; but they can do nothing whatever in surgery, even in the simplest cases : if anything at all is attempted, it is almost sure to be the reverse of what ought to be done. In the skilful practice of surgery ,therefore, the medical missionary's influence will be most felt and appreciated, and to this department, while a student, he ought to give very special attention.

It is not, however, to the professional training of the medical missionary that we here refer; we may leave this with perfect confidence to our universities and medical schools, and accept the medical and surgical diplomas which they grant as satisfactory evidence that he is, professionally, fully qualified for his work. The success of the medical missionary is not to be estimated by his fame as a physician or surgeon, except in so far as he has grace and wisdom to use the influence thus acquired for the promotion of the great object in view— success will show itself in his being wise to win souls. Not every Christian physician, therefore, is qualified for the work of a medical missionary. The cause has suffered not a little from so-called medical missionaries having been sent forth to the mission field—men who have had no special training for the work, and have possessed no special evangelistic gift.

The training of the medical missionary must, to a large extent, be practical. He must be a devout believer, holding with a firm and intelligent grasp the saving truths of the Gospel, a thoughtful student of the Bible, and possessed of evangelistic gifts; such a man may surely be trusted to preach to the heathen the simple truths of Christianity, without any special systematic instruction in the technicalities and controversies of theological science. Much wisdom and care should, however, be exercised in the selection for training of young men who are desirous of devoting themselves to this work. Added to sound health, good mental ability, enthusiastic love of the profession, and, above all, evidence of the constraining influence of the love of Christ, one other qualification is essential, namely, the possession of the gifts and graces needed to make them successful evangelists; and during their course of study, they should have every opportunity, under proper superintendence, for acquiring experience, in combining their professional work with judicious but zealous evangelistic effort. This is the aim and object of the training institution in connection with the Edinburgh Medical Missionary Society; and we can desire no better evidence of the value of the practical medico-evangelistic training there enjoyed by the medical missionary students, than the successful work accomplished by those who have gone forth from the institution, and are now occupying spheres of influence and usefulness in the mission field, all over the world.

Another question of great practical importance calls for consideration. Some friends of the cause think that medical missionaries should be allowed to better their circumstances either by engaging, to a limited extent, in private practice, where opportunities for such practice exist, or, that they should receive a higher rate of salary than ordinary missionaries.

To both of these proposals we most emphatically object. The one implies, on the part of the medical missionary, a half-hearted consecration to the work, and has given rise to no end of difficulties; the other, that he possesses certain gifts and qualifications which may, under certain circumstances, give him greater opportunities for usefulness, and that he ought therefore to be more highly remunerated. Such a principle, if acted upon, would strike at the root of missionary consecration abroad, and quench the true missionary spirit at home. The medical missionary goes forth, not from worldly motives, not for the sake of salary, but for his Master's sake, rejoicing in this, that if his acquirements gain for him a greater influence, and a readier access to the households of the heathen, he enjoys all the higher privilege in being permitted to consecrate such gifts and graces upon the missionary altar.

When a medical missionary goes out to India, or to China, two paths are open before him—the path of worldly advancement and profit, and the path of self-sacrifice and consecration to his special work. If he yield to the temptation to cultivate a select, private practice, or to accept some lucrative appointment, he may soon secure for himself a good income; but, in doing so, let him clearly understand that he is turning aside from his proper work, and is applying to his special department of service a principle which, if applied to other departments, as with equal justice it might be, would speedily bring the missionary enterprise into contempt.

On this point, in a paper on " Medical Missions," read
at a missionary conference in Japan, Dr. John C. Berry,
of the American Board of Commissioners for Foreign
Missions, says :

"I must here call attention to an evil which has,
in too many instances, embarrassed the efforts and
weakened the influence of medical missionaries. I refer
to the too prevalent custom of engaging in private
practice among the foreign residents at the open ports,
where there are established medical men. The practice
is unjust to the physician, to the patients, to ourselves,
and, in an inexpressible degree, to the general interests of
our work ;—to the physician, in unfairly competing with
him, and depriving him of much of his legitimate income ; to the patients, who, in learning to look to us as
their family physician, are obliged, during our absence
on frequent tours, to receive the professional services of
another, who may know nothing of the constitutional
peculiarities of the family ; to ourselves, in burdening us
with additional cares, and depriving us of that deep sense
of satisfaction which an extended and prosperous work
on purely mission lines affords ; and to the general
interests of the work, in that it takes from it very much
valuable time, constantly introduces to our notice a work
which tends to weaken our sympathy with missionary
effort, and awakens in the minds, both of the resident
foreigners and native people, a suspicion of our personal
disinterestedness and entire devotion to the cause."

The position which we have indicated as that which the medical missionary should occupy, can only be filled by one separated for the work by God Himself. Contemplating this work, grand alike in its medical and missionary aspects, we may well exclaim, "Who is sufficient for these things?" The reply of the true medical missionary will be, "Our sufficiency is of God." In his experience it holds true, as in the experience of all whom God calls into His service, "to him that hath shall be given."

We cannot perhaps better illustrate what we believe to be the proper sphere and function of the medical missionary, than by offering a few hints suggested by our own experience of medical missionary work in India.

During his first year in India, China, or elsewhere, the medical missionary ought to devote his chief time and attention to the acquisition of the language. If possible, he should reside during that period with an experienced missionary, at some distance from the station where he expects eventually to establish his medical mission, but where the same language is spoken. Unless some such arrangement is made, he will soon find himself burdened with the anxieties of a large practice, which will sadly interfere with his linguistic studies. We attach so much importance to the first year being kept almost entirely free for the study of the language, that we strongly recommend that his full medical and surgical outfit should not be supplied till he has passed his examination in the

vernacular. Experience proves that if at the close of
the first year a good beginning has not been made in the
acquisition of the language, after progress is very slow,
and the missionary's usefulness suffers irreparably during
his whole future course.

Having acquired some degree of fluency in the use
of the language, he should open his dispensary in as
central a locality as possible. From the first he should,
if practicable, associate with himself an earnest, intelligent, judicious native evangelist—not with the view of
delegating to another his evangelistic duties, but for the
purpose of following up, thoroughly and systematically,
his own spiritual ministrations. In his visits the native
evangelist should accompany him, and in all his labours
he should be closely identified with him. As the work
goes on, the medical missionary will lose sight of many of
his patients, who, no longer needing his advice, pass away
from his observation and influence; but these the native
evangelist should follow to their homes and regularly
visit, and, as a rule, he will always be gladly welcomed.

At the dispensary, in commencing the work of the
day, the medical missionary should himself address the
patients and their friends assembled in the waiting-room,
and conduct a short service with them. The native
evangelist should, however, be present, and, while the
cases are being examined, he should make sure that no
one shall leave without having been personally dealt
with, and directed to the Great Physician for spiritual

healing. By taking advantage in this way of native help, a vast amount of most hopeful evangelistic work may be daily accomplished, and much permanent fruit be gathered in.

Two or three intelligent native Christian youths should as soon as possible be selected and trained as assistants. They will soon be able to dispense medicines, serve as dressers, and do all the drudgery of dispensary work, and thus much of the medical missionary's time will be set free for more important duties. Whatever he can train his native assistants to do as well as he can himself, ought never, as a rule, to occupy his time and attention. In training his native assistants, Bible reading, exposition, and prayer should inaugurate each day's teaching and work, and he ought constantly to impress upon their minds that their highest aim should ever be the spiritual welfare of the patients.

He should, as soon as circumstances permit, open a hospital, on a small scale at first—perhaps only providing accommodation for two or three patients, but gradually increasing the number of beds as funds are forthcoming and the need arises.  It is in the hospital that the most satisfactory and successful medical and surgical work will be accomplished—work which will produce the deepest impression, and direct public attention most favourably to the higher objects of the mission.  It is here, too, that the medical missionary will be able most successfully to accomplish evangelistic work—here that he may expect to gather the most precious and enduring fruit. While dispensary work, and occasionally medico-evangelistic tours among the surrounding towns and villages, are important features of medical missionary work, still the hospital will be the field in which the richest harvest will be reaped, and therefore the establishment of a hospital should from the first be kept in view, and accomplished at the earliest opportunity.

The medical care of the missionaries and their families will form no small nor unimportant part of his duties, but, with this exception, the medical missionary should have as little as possible to do with practice among Europeans ; he should certainly decline such practice where other medical aid can be obtained, and while ready, under other circumstances, to stretch forth the helping hand whenever and wherever his aid may be needed, he will never fail to put the disinterestedness of his motives beyond all suspicion by placing to the credit of the mission whatever fees he may receive.

While his time will generally be well occupied in attending to his own special department of work, still, by taking full advantage of native help, he will, by and by, find both time and opportunity for promoting, in co-operation with his ministerial colleagues, schemes for the physical, social, and intellectual improvement of the people, and occasionally for more or less extended medico-evangelistic tours.

It is of the utmost importance that harmony should

5

exist between the medical missionary and his ministerial
colleagues, and in order to maintain this, both must
esteem each other very highly for their works' sake, must
consult one with another, and manifest mutual sympathy
in all that pertains to their respective spheres of labour.
There must be perfect equality, perfect confidence, and
hearty co-operation. They must look upon the work in
all its departments as one, and work hand in hand in all
their efforts. Carried on in this spirit, and on the lines
which we have indicated, the value of medical missions
can hardly be over-estimated.

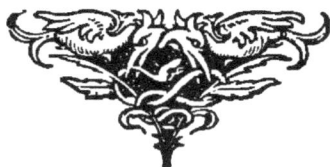

# THE VALUE OF MEDICAL MISSIONS AS A PIONEER AGENCY

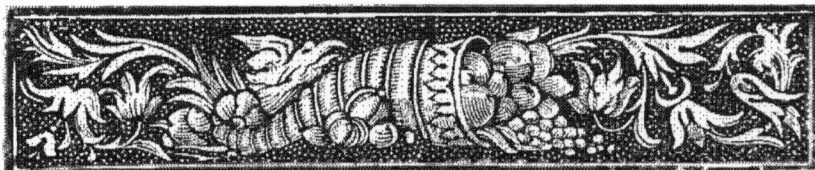

## CHAPTER III.

The value of Medical Missions as a Pioneer Agency; the Testimony of Travellers, and the Experience of Missionaries.

AS a means of overcoming prejudice, and of gaining access to heathen, and often exclusive, communities, medical missions present strong claims to the sympathy and support of the friends of missions. The suspicion and prejudice with which the Christian missionary is often regarded in Mohammedan countries, as well as in many parts of the heathen world, render our endeavours to reach the people, and introduce the Gospel amongst them, a work of great difficulty, and often even of danger. Gross ignorance, superstition, and fanaticism, caste, social habits, and national prejudices, are barriers which the mere missionary finds it difficult to overcome, and which may compel him to remain for years isolated

and shunned, if not despised, and thus the opportunity
of doing good for which he yearns is utterly denied him ;
whilst, to the missionary physician, the hovel and the
palace are alike opened at his approach, suspicions are
allayed, prejudice is disarmed, caste distinction, for the
time at least, is overcome ; even the harem, where the
brother may not intrude, is not too sacred for the
" infidel " when he enters as an angel of mercy to the
sick and dying : thus, as the missionary pioneer, he
opens and holds open many a door of Christian usefulness—to these he introduces his brethren, thus enlarging
their sphere of service as well as his own.

Sir Henry Halford, late President of the Royal College
of Physicians, in an address on " The Results of the
Successful Practice of Physic " delivered many years ago
to the college, related an interesting historical fact from
which he deduced an important practical lesson. " A
circumstance," Sir Henry said, " most flattering to the
medical profession is the establishment of the East India
Company's power on the coast of Coromandel, procured
from the Great Mogul in gratitude for the efficient help
of Dr. Gabriel Boughton in a case of great distress. It
seems that in the year 1636 one of the princesses of the
imperial family had been dreadfully burnt, and a messenger was sent to Surat to desire the assistance of one
of the English surgeons there, when Boughton proceeded
forthwith to Delhi, and performed the cure. On the
minister of the Great Mogul asking him what his master

could do for him to manifest his gratitude for so important a service, Boughton answered, with a disinterestedness, a generosity, and a patriotism beyond all praise, 'Let my nation trade with yours.' 'Be it so,' was the reply. A portion of the coast was marked out for the resort of English ships, and all duties were compromised for a small sum of money. Here did the civilization of that vast continent commence—and hence the blessed light of the Gospel began to be promulgated among the millions of idolaters, since subjugated to the control of the British power. This happy result of the successful interposition of one of our medical brethren suggests to my mind the question of the expediency of educating missionaries in the medical art. I am sanguine enough to believe that even the proud and exclusive Chinese would receive those who entered their country with these views without suspicion or distrust, which they never fail to manifest when they surmise that trade is the object of the strangers' visit or some covert intention to interfere with their institutions."

Another instance of the happy influence exerted by the professional services of a British surgeon occurred in 1713—when the success of an embassy of complaint, sent by the Presidency of Bengal to the Court of Delhi was mainly due to Mr. Hamilton, surgeon of the embassy, having cured a painful disease with which the Emperor was afflicted. Mr. Hamilton was offered any reward he chose to ask, and he generously confined himself to requesting the Emperor's compliance with the demands of the embassy, which was instantly granted ; and thus privileges of the greatest importance were obtained which enabled the East India Company to establish their possessions on a sure basis.

From a worldly point of view, how vast are the results which have flowed from the skill and disinterestedness of these men ; and what the love of their profession and their patriotism led them to do for their country, might surely be accomplished by the missionary physician, who goes forth, impelled by the love of Christ, to heal the sick and to preach the Gospel.   In his " Hints on Missions," published so long ago as 1822, Mr. Douglas of Cavers writes :  " If with scientific attainments missionaries combined the profession of physic, it would be attended with many advantages ; for there is something suspicious in a foreigner remaining long in a country without an openly defined object which the people can appreciate.   The character of a physician has always been highly honoured in the East, and would give an easy and unsuspected admission to familiar intercourse with all classes and creeds.   He who is a physician is pardoned for being a Christian, religious and national prejudices disappear before him, all hearts and harems are opened, and he is welcomed as if he were carrying to the dying the elixir of immortality."

The experience of travellers and of missionaries everywhere, bears emphatic testimony to the value of medical missions as a pioneer agency. The late Dr. Asahel Grant is described, among the Nestorians, as armed with his needle and lancet for the removal of cataract, forcing mountain passes which the sword could never penetrate, and in the wilds of the Nestorian mountains, and amid ferocious warriors, winning his way to their homes and hearts, and traversing in safety regions hitherto untrodden by civilized man.

Fortune, in his work entitled " Residence among the Chinese," bears the following testimony :—

" The Chinese," he says, " are, as a nation, jealous, selfish, and eminently conceited ; it is difficult, therefore, to convince such minds that nations, many thousand miles distant, will subscribe large sums of money merely for their religious benefit; or that men are to be found who will leave friends and home, with no other object in view than to convert them to Christianity. Hence it would seem that the labours of the medical missionary prove a powerful auxiliary in aiding the spread of the Gospel among such a people. All nations, even the most cold and selfish, have some kindly feelings in their nature capable of being roused and acted upon; and if anything will warm such feelings in the mind of the Chinese, the labour of the medical missionary is well calculated to do so. The blind receive their sight, the lame walk, and the wounded and diseased are cured ; and thus, when the better feelings are expanded into something like gratitude, prejudices are more likely to give way, and the mind may become softened and more receptive of religious impressions."

In confirmation of such independent testimony, there is no lack of evidence from missionaries themselves. " My own experience," writes the Rev. H. Corbett, "and so far as I know, that of all missionaries, in China, agree in this, that one of the greatest obstacles in preaching to the heathen is the prejudice and suspicion which is everywhere encountered, and the medical missionary has a power to overcome this difficulty possessed by no other agency. In connection with our mission in the south, in some cases, every attempt to get a hold in a new city failed, until the medical missionary first won the confidence of the people by healing, or at least relieving, cases beyond the skill of the native physician. The preacher, known to be the friend of the doctor, then met with a welcome; and flourishing churches, with native pastors, have since been formed in more than one city and town in which the work was thus begun. The same, I believe, is true of other parts of China. In the present stage of the work, I am persuaded that well qualified medical missionaries are indispensable to the efficiency and success of the work here."

Some time ago, the Directors of the Edinburgh Medical Missionary Society received an urgent appeal for a medical missionary, signed by seven missionaries in connection with the American Presbyterian Mission in China. "Medical work in China," they say, "has been one of the most fruitful departments of missionary labour. It has diffused a knowledge of civilization, removed prejudice, and conciliated goodwill more than any other agency. Our missionary work has been greatly retarded because, hitherto, medical work has not been connected with it; hence we are anxious that this important auxiliary should be at once supplied."

Dr. Parker, through whose instrumentality the Edinburgh Medical Missionary Society was formed, and whose long experience of medical missionary work in China gives weight to his testimony, says : "I have no hesitation in expressing it as my solemn conviction that, as yet, no medium of contact, and of bringing the people under the sound of the Gospel, and within the influence of other means of grace, can compare with the facilities afforded by medical missionary operations."

A striking illustration of the value of medical missionary work is the providential opening for the establishment of a medical mission at Tientsin which occurred in 1879. During the visit to Tientsin of Dr. Mackenzie, a medical missionary of the London Missionary Society at Hankow, Lady Li, wife of His Excellency Li Hung-Chang, the Governor-General of the Province, who had been long an invalid, was so dangerously ill, that her native physicians had given her up. They told the Governor-General that they could do nothing more for her, except to begin and give over again all the drugs which had already been administered! In this emergency, his Excellency, having

heard of the visit of Dr. Mackenzie to the city, summoned him, along with Dr. Irwin, to attend Lady Li
As Chinese prejudice forbids much that is allowed to
Occidental practice, it was found necessary to call in a
lady physician. Miss L. H. Howard, M.D., of the
American Methodist Mission, was providentially at no
great distance from Tientsin, and having been sent for,
she was soon installed in a suite of rooms in the official
residence, adjoining her ladyship's apartments. With
God's blessing on the treatment of these three physicians,
added to careful nursing, Lady Li's life was saved, and
she was soon quite restored to health. The fame of
foreign medicine was in this way quickly spread abroad,
and received the highest approval. The physicians had
soon plenty of work. While they remained in the Yamen,
or official residence, they operated successfully in many
serious surgical cases, and as native doctors know nothing
of surgery, the wonderful cures effected produced a great
impression. The Governor-General fitted up a dispensary
for Dr. Mackenzie in a temple—the largest in Tientsin,
built as a memorial to his predecessor—furnished the
medicines, and allowed him full liberty to preach the
Gospel to his patients. Accommodation was likewise provided, in another part of the same temple, for Miss Dr.
Howard's dispensary for women, his Excellency paying
all expenses, and granting to her the same privilege.
Thousands of Chinese, including all classes of society,
came to these dispensaries for medical aid, and had

the Gospel preached to them, humanly speaking, under the most favourable circumstances; and so great was the encouragement in this work, that, on the invitation of his Excellency, Dr. Mackenzie determined to remain permanently at Tientsin.  A difficulty, however, soon presented itself: the temple, which was used as a dispensary and hospital, was three miles distant from the foreign settlement, and Dr. Mackenzie found it quite impossible, at that distance, to give proper attention to his patients, especially in serious surgical cases.  With the sanction of the Viceroy, who promised to contribute handsomely to the building fund, it was accordingly determined to erect an in-patient hospital in a more convenient locality.   About this time Dr. Mackenzie rendered valuable medical help to General Chow, who forthwith presented five hundred taels (£150) for the benefit of the hospital.   This timely gift suggested the idea of sending a subscription list to other wealthy Chinese officials, and liberal contributions flowed in.  A substantial and commodious hospital was built, and at the opening ceremony, his Excellency the Viceroy graced the occasion by his presence, and expressed the pleasure he had in taking part in a work such as they were inaugurating. The medical mission has since then been carried on with uninterrupted success, and many have received through its instrumentality the "double cure," and in the city evangelistic work has been most successfully prosecuted. Much interest attaches to this work in Tientsin, all the necessary funds for its support being obtained from native sources. "It is a new thing," writes the Rev. Griffith John, "for the Chinese to tolerate the propagation of Christian tenets in connection with institutions established and supported by themselves; it must be that they are beginning to look on the Gospel in a new light, and that some of their old prejudices are gradually melting away."

A young medical missionary, Dr. H. N. Allen, was during the past year sent by the American Presbyterian Board to Corea. He proceeded with fear and trembling, scarcely knowing whether he would be even admitted; but he found himself welcomed by all classes. Soon after, upon the occasion of a violent political outbreak, he was placed in charge of some scores of wounded men, mainly of high rank and representing the contending parties. He was the means of saving the life of Min Yong Ik, the nephew of the king, and the head of the embassy which some months ago visited America. Dr. Allen has been, by these remarkable providences, raised to a position of great influence. When all the foreigners, including the diplomatic representatives of Europe and America, were compelled to flee to the coast, he with his wife and child remained alone at the capital, where they were shielded by the influence which as a physician he possessed. The military forces of the king were placed as a guard around his house, and accompanied him on his visits to his patients. As an expression of gratitude for his services, the Government now propose to provide him with a hospital for his work.

The prince whose life he had saved said to him, " Our people cannot believe that you came from America ; they insist that you must have dropped from heaven for this special crisis." When Dr. Allen was called to Min Yong Ik, he found thirteen native doctors trying to staunch his wounds by filling them with wax. Standing aside for the young missionary, they looked on with amazement, while he tied the arteries and sewed up the gaping wounds. Thus in a few minutes a revolution was effected in the medical treatment of the kingdom, at the same time an incalculable vantage-ground was thus gained for the introduction of the Gospel.

There is perhaps no better instance of the value of medical missions as a pioneer agency, than the remarkable success of the medical mission in connection with the Church Missionary Society in Kashmir. Before medical mission work was tried in Kashmir, the Rev. Messrs. Clark and Smith, two of the most experienced of the C. M. S. missionaries, had gone with six native preachers to break ground there, but were soon driven out of the valley. Dr. Elmslie was then sent to commence a medical mission, and, with God's blessing, succeeded in opening the door which had hitherto been closed, and by his medical skill he thus gained an entrance for himself and his brother missionaries to one of the greatest strongholds of heathenism in India. The late Lord Bishop of Calcutta (the Right Rev. Dr. Cotton) when in Kashmir visited the dispensary, and thus refers to the good work carried on there : " It is but little that we can at present do to make known to the Kashmiris the blessings of Christ's salvation ; but I quite believe that Dr. Elmslie is knocking at the one door which may, through God's help, be opened for the truth to enter in. The scene appeared to me most interesting and edifying, and could not fail to remind me of Him who ' went about all Galilee preaching the Gospel of the kingdom, and healing all manner of sickness and disease among the people.' "

During the late Afghan war, the fierce Wuziri mountaineers made a rush upon and sacked the town of Tank, on the extreme border of British territory. At this place the Church Missionary Society has a medical mission, carried on by the Rev. John Williams, a native doctor and clergyman, whose influence with the Afghan population throughout a wide district had always been very great. The wild, fierce-looking Wuziris had learned to look upon John Williams as their kind and good friend, and when they swept down from their mountain fastnesses they spared the C. M. S. Mission Hospital and premises.

The London Missionary Society's Medical Mission in Travancore has been a most valuable auxiliary to evangelistic work in that Province. In the waiting-room of the mission dispensary may be seen, day by day, sitting side by side under the same roof, the Brahmin, Súdra, and Shānar, the Pulayar and Pariah, the devil-worshipper and the follower of Siva, the Mohammedan, Roman Catholic, and Protestant Christian—men, women, and children of all castes and creeds, waiting their turn to be examined, and listening attentively to the reading of God's Word and the preaching of the Gospel. There, year by year, thousands hear the sweet story of redeeming love, who would otherwise, in all human probability, live and die without having once had an opportunity of listening to the glad tidings.

Shortly before the writer retired from the superintendence of the medical mission in Travancore, there lived together for nearly two months in the same ward of the hospital a young Brahmin and his mother ; a Súdra, his wife, and brother ; and a Shānar boy and his mother. The Brahmin youth had a compound fracture of the right leg, and a simple fracture of the left leg ; the Súdra had fracture of the skull, with a severe scalp wound ; and the Shānar boy had a compound fracture of the thigh, and simple fracture of both arms, the result of a fall from a palmyra tree. For the time being, at least, broken bones levelled caste distinction, and created a bond of sympathy between them. As a physician, in visiting the sick at their homes, we had peculiar facilities for reaching a class otherwise very inaccessible, and of commending the truth not only to our patients, but also to the large crowds of villagers which thronged around us. An entrance was

6

thus gained into communities, and a welcome access obtained to the homes of caste families, which would probably have remained closed to the visits of the ordinary missionary.

By means of his medical skill exercised in the successful treatment of the Rance—wife of the Maharajah—Dr. Colin Valentine gained access, both for himself and his brother missionaries, to Jeypore, one of the most bigoted and exclusive strongholds of idolatry in Northern India, where the United Presbyterian Church has now a prosperous mission. Dr. Valentine was at first stationed at Beawr, in the state of Mairwarra. His health, however, broke down, and he was ordered to go to the Himalayas for rest and change. On his way he had to pass through Jeypore, and while there he visited the Maharajah, who told him, in the course of conversation, that one of his favourite Ranees was very ill, that the native doctors could do nothing for her, and that he would be very glad if he would see her. Dr. Valentine at once consented, and, under very difficult circumstances, succeeded in diagnosing the nature of the Ranee's illness. By the blessing of God on the means used, she was restored to health. Previous to this, no missionary had been allowed to settle in that native state. After the recovery of the Rance, overtures were made to Dr. Valentine to remain at Jeypore as his Highness's physician ; he at once told the Maharajah that he was a missionary, and that unless he were allowed to carry on missionary work without let or hindrance, however high the position, he could not possibly accept it. The condition was accepted by his Highness, and Dr. Valentine remained at Jeypore for fourteen years ; and thus, by the Divine blessing on the medical mission agency, the native state and city of Jeypore were opened up to the Gospel of Christ.

The Rev. Mr. Ellis, in his deeply interesting narrative of the triumphs of the Gospel in Madagascar, thus refers to the influence of the medical department there : "The dispensary, which Dr. Davidson opened as soon as practicable after his arrival, has been for some time in successful operation. The assistance rendered to the sick, and the skill with which the doctor had treated a large proportion of the multitude who daily sought his help, deeply impressed the inhabitants of the capital and the suburbs. The cure in some cases, and relief in others from long standing and, in their circumstances, hopeless suffering which so many experienced, was regarded with great satisfaction by all residing within reach of the dispensary. But the fame of the cures effected spread far beyond those who had experienced these benefits ; and of the vast number of strangers who throng the capital, few return to their homes without paying a visit to the dispensary, to witness the benefits conferred upon others or to seek relief for themselves. In addition to the usefulness of dispensary in alleviating physical suffering, it exercises a powerful influence for good as an auxiliary to our mission. It is a standing testimony to the beneficence of our Divine religion, and is calculated to impress upon the people a more just appreciation of the value of human life than has hitherto, unfortunately, prevailed. It has, to no inconsiderable extent, disarmed the prejudices and conciliated the affections of the people. Its influence in this respect has been felt among all classes, from the sovereign downwards. It has done more : it has brought the Gospel to a large class who could not possibly be reached by any other agency whatever. Many have listened to the Gospel for the first time in the mission dispensary, where they have resorted for the cure of their bodily ailments, whose enmity and indifference would have prevented them seeking or even submitting to counsel or instruction from any other source."

Another striking illustration of the influence of the missionary physician is the successful work carried on at Urambo, Central Africa, by the late lamented Dr. Southon, of the London Missionary Society. Dr. Southon, on his way to join the missionaries at Ujiji, had to pass through Urambo. Mirambo, the king, hearing that the new missionary was a doctor, sent messengers with the request that he would visit him, and relieve him of a painful tumour on his arm. Dr. Southon proceeded to Urambo, saw the king, and at once proposed to remove the tumour. Chloroform was administered, and the operation successfully performed. The king, very grateful for the relief afforded, earnestly requested Dr. Southon to remain at Urambo, and es--

tablish a mission at the capital, promised to build him a house and hospital, to provide everything necessary for his comfort as well as for the work, and to give him as much land as he needed. "The country is before you," he said : "choose where you will, it is all yours." Dr. Southon selected a very luxuriant hill near by, where a good spring of water and plenty of trees made it a very desirable station, and henceforth his letters were dated from " Calton Hill," Urambo. He succeeded in establishing a most hopeful mission ; his relations with Mirambo continued friendly till the last, and he won for himself the confidence of the people. The seeds of Divine truth were sown broadcast, and when he was so suddenly and mysteriously cut down in the midst of his usefulness, there was bitter mourning among the Wanyamwezi, and none manifested more profound grief than did King Mirambo.

The great evangelistic problem yet to be solved is, how aggressive missionary work can be best promoted among Mohammedan and Jewish communities. It has been well said, "The more of truth there is in any false or defective system of religion, the harder will be the task of those who seek to displace or supplant it by the presentation of the truth as it is in Jesus; and as Jew and Mohammedan alike firmly hold the great truth of the unity of the Godhead, it becomes very difficult to persuade them that there is a Trinity in unity, and that God sent His Son to be the Saviour of the world.

Hence the absolute need of the most thoroughly scriptural presentation of the Gospel to people with opinions firmly rooted in truth." And what more scriptural presentation of the Gospel could be devised than that enjoined by the Master, when He gave His commission to the seventy : " Heal the sick, and say unto them, The kingdom of God is come nigh unto you."

Lieut. Van de Velde, Dutch R.N., in his "Narrative of a Journey through Syria and Palestine," thus speaks of the difficulties of missionary work in the East, and of the value of medical missions : " A great hindrance to missionary labour here, arises from the difficulty of finding access to the people. The bitter hatred entertained by the Rabbis toward a living Christianity, and, in particular, towards the missionaries, makes it almost impossible for the latter to speak to the Jews about the concerns of their souls. On this account, the London Society has very wisely attached to its agency at Jerusalem a Medical Mission, where gratuitous attendance is given to the sick. The haughty heart, when broken by the disease of the body, is willing to listen to the voice of Divine compassion, especially when the lips of those from whom that voice proceeds are in correspondence with the benevolent hand of human sympathy and tenderness. This is the way pointed out to us by the Lord Jesus Christ Himself—the way which, methinks, is too much neglected by missionaries and missionary societies."

In the course of his journey homewards from

Bokhara, the Rev. Dr. Wolff passed through Damascus, and saw Dr. Thompson, a medical missionary of the Syrian Medical Aid Association, at work there. In his account of his travels, he testifies to Dr. Thompson's remarkable success in winning the regard and esteem of the bigoted Mohammedan population around. "I am deeply convinced," he says, "that incalculable benefit has been conferred on the eastern world by the mission of Dr. Thompson, for I have learned, not only from Europeans, but also from Armenians and Turks, how zealously and successfully he has been engaged at Damascus. I am sure that medical men as missionaries would most powerfully subserve the promotion of Christianity in the East."

After labouring some years in Damascus, Dr. Thompson was removed to Antioch, and shortly after settling there he wrote: "Immediately on my arrival here my services were in requisition. I was before known to the chief Turkish families in this place, and though Antioch is considered one of the great strong-holds of Moslem fanaticism and Jewish obstinacy, still, I am truly thankful to say, I never was in a place where I have met with more kindness, and such an apparently sincere desire on the part of all to give me a hearty greeting. They know of my services in years past in Damascus, Aleppo Beyrout, &c., and therefore they are all prepared to avail themselves of my aid in times of need. It is not unusual for me to be accosted in the streets by people of

all ranks, and requested to feel the pulse, and suggest
something to remove some trifling ailment ; this begets a
friendly intercourse. Mrs. Thompson is invited to the
*harems* of the Turks, and she can walk unmolested
through the bazaars, though it is quite a new thing to
the people to see a European lady going about thus."

The Rev. Mr. Knapp, who, with Dr. Haskell as his
medical colleague, laboured long and successfully in
Central Turkey, in pleading for the addition of a medical
missionary to the staff of the mission at Bitlis, thus
expresses himself: "Here, a missionary who is a physician will have access to a far greater number than he
could possibly reach were he not a physician, and this
is emphatically true in opening new fields of labour.
The greatest solicitude the missionary has, in such places,
is to get a hearing. Men will not come to him, nor will
they receive him if he goes to them. Now, the physician draws the people to himself. Men naturally care
more for their bodies than for their souls, and in this
country they have a high, almost a superstitious, regard
for a ' Frank' educated physician. One day a Mussulman called upon us, and begged for a ' bit of bread.' On
inquiry, we learned that he wanted it to give to his
brother, who was lying sick of a fever, and we found he
had the notion that a few crumbs of the ' Frank's' bread
would cure him ! At first we thought it a mere farce,
and would have turned him away as imposing upon us,
but his continued entreaties convinced us that he was in

earnest. This was before Dr. Haskell arrived, and I
mention this incident to show what unbounded confidence such a people would be likely to place, and in
fact do place, in a missionary physician. He is called
everywhere the 'hakem bashe' (the great physician),
and he will not only have access to those in the town in
which he resides, but many from surrounding villages
will come to him, who would never think of visiting a
simple missionary. So far as our observation goes, we
can safely affirm that here the medical missionary has
ten times more access to the people than the ordinary
missionary."

Reference has already been made to Dr. Grant's
work. Patients thronged from all parts to get his advice;
many were carried by friends as many as five days'
journey. Nestorians came from the mountains, Kurdish
chiefs even from Amadia beyond, and some from the
distant borders of Georgia. Among his patients were
many of the highest rank and influence—princes of the
royal family, governors of provinces, and many of the
Persian nobility, and he never failed to avail himself of
the opportunities thus afforded of sowing broadcast the
seeds of Divine truth. Writing to the secretary of the
society whose honoured agent he was, Dr. Grant says :
" As I have witnessed the relief of hitherto hopeless
suffering, and seen their grateful attempts to kiss my
feet, and my very shoes at the door, both of which they
would literally bathe with tears—especially as I have seen

the haughty Moolah stoop to kiss the border of the despised Christian, thanking God that I would not refuse medicine to a Moslem, and others saying that in every prayer they thanked God for my coming. I have felt that, even before I could teach our religion, I was doing something to recommend it and to break down prejudices, and wished that more of my professional brethren might share the luxury of doing such work for Christ."

On the death of Dr. Grant, his colleague thus wrote concerning his work: " Dr. Grant had twenty times more intercourse with the Mohammedans than the missionary sent out expressly to labour amongst them. No European had hitherto resided in this remote Persian town (Urumiah), and the rude and bloody character of its Mussulman inhabitants was so notorious, that our English friends at Tabrez deemed our enterprise extremely hazardous. Dr. Grant was the man for the place and the period; his skilful practice as a physician soon won the respect and confidence of all classes, and contributed very materially to our security, and to the permanent success of our mission—more, doubtless, than any other earthly means."

The Rev. Robert Bruce, the well-known missionary of the Church Missionary Society in Persia, appealing for a medical associate, thus wrote to us: " My object in writing at present is to ask your kind assistance in obtaining, what is the great desideratum of our mission, a medical missionary for Persia. Edinburgh is, I believe, the best place to look for one, and I cannot but believe that, if the great wants of Persia, and the splendid field which is here open to a medical missionary, were made known, we should soon find one ready to volunteer for the work. Surely medical missionaries are more needed in Mohammedan lands than anywhere. A medical missionary would have at once a noble field open for him both in Julfa and Ispahan, plenty, and not too much, work, a most intelligent and interesting people to work among, and a splendid climate. A medical missionary could reside in Ispahan, in the centre of the Mohammedan population, and, most probably, would prepare the way for an ordained missionary taking up his residence there, which is impossible at present. May God make use of these words, and choose a man Himself." In response to this appeal, Dr. Hœrnle, one of the students of the Edinburgh Medical Missionary Society, offered his services to the Church Missionary Society, and since 1879 has been labouring with much success in Ispahan.

The success of the work carried on by Dr. Vartan, in connection with the Edinburgh Medical Missionary Society's hospital and dispensary at Nazareth, is a striking illustration of the value of this agency in a Mohammedan community. Out of one hundred and seventy-five indoor patients treated during the year, there were one hundred and sixteen Moslems, twenty-nine Greeks, twenty Roman Catholics, and one Druse. The average length of time each patient remained in the hospital was twenty-nine days, and during that time each of these received daily Christian instruction. During the same period, upwards of six thousand patients came to the dispensary for advice, and of these there was about the same proportion of Moslems, Greeks, Roman Catholics, and Protestants. A few incidents of the daily work carried on amongst the patients, both indoor and outdoor, may be alike interesting and instructive.

One day there happened to be present in the waiting-room about half a dozen Bedouins, real children of the desert. They sat together, rather uncomfortably, in the middle of the room, seemingly very much encumbered with their swords and pistol-cases. They had come to get advice and medicine, but they could not understand why so many all round the room were sitting so quietly, or, if talking with their neighbours, doing so in a low voice. To do them credit, they tried to behave like the others, but they were evidently unaccustomed to restrain their feelings. It was still more puzzling to them to see the doctor coming in, opening a book, reading from it, and then speaking to the congregation. They looked at first as if they had made a mistake ; they glanced at each other and seemed to say, "This cannot be the place to which we were directed to come for medicine ;" and if they could, they would have risen and gone out, but they were surrounded by patients, and could not leave. By and by they settled down, listened very attentively, and seemed to understand something of the address. The doctor was speaking about the solemnity of the Day of Judgment, and urging the necessity for preparation for that great day. One, the eldest of the Bedouin group, turned round and said audibly to his companions, "When that time comes, I will ride on my swift mare, and be off to the desert." This remark caused the others to laugh, when an old sheikh from among the patients stood up and gravely rebuked them, reminding them at the same time of the seriousness of the subject. The interruption was short, and the doctor continued his address, and these poor Bedouins, as well as all the others, were assured that none could escape by any efforts of their own ; that they need not fear the approach of that day if they would but "behold the Lamb of God which taketh away the sin of the world."

On another occasion, just as the doctor was beginning the short service, there came stepping in a great Moslem chief, with half a dozen attendants. A little commotion was observed among the assembled patients and their friends, but it was only to clear the best part of the room for the distinguished visitor, who took the place so kindly offered to him. He was very attentive during the whole service, but was startled more than once when some point contrary to his religion was touched upon, and two or three times he audibly exclaimed, "There is no god but God"—an expression often used as a spell to prevent one from being influenced when Christ is spoken of as the Son of God ; but before the service was over he seemed quite interested, and when he came into the consulting-room he said to the doctor, " Surely the Bible from which you have been reading to us is not the Bible that was used in the time of Mohammed, for, if it had presented Christ—as you in your address said that it does —as the Eternal Word and the Eternal Son, co-existent with the Father, and not related as men are on earth, Mohammed would not, I think, have condemned it as he did." He was assured that it was the same, but that human tradition had corrupted Christianity, both in the time of Mohammed and in our own time. He asked for a Bible, that he might read it carefully for himself. He received a copy, and now diligently studies the Word of God. May the Divine Spirit enlighten his understanding !

"Some native friends advised me," writes Dr. Vartan, "since the spread of the news of the late disturbances, to suspend the religious services for a time, lest my congregation, being chiefly Mohammedans, some of them fanatics, should make it a pretext to excite mischief. We thanked them for their counsel, but resolved to make no change ; and not only has nothing unpleasant happened, but my Mohammedan audience is as quiet and respectful as hitherto. Indeed, in many cases, they are even more attentive and more reverential during the prayers than many so-called Christians, and, I may add, more grateful for services rendered to them. We find here, both among

Mohammedans and Greeks, that the Word of God is not hindered by any material force, but that it is only the hardening of man's heart that keeps the Heavenly Guest waiting outside."

In the hospital, always the most hopeful and satisfactory sphere of labour in connection with a medical mission, much precious seed has been sown, and not a little fruit has been gathered. The patients are kindly and lovingly dealt with, and all, while inmates of the hospital, receive regular Christian instruction; indeed, it would be almost impossible for any one to remain in it, for any length of time, without obtaining some knowledge of the fundamental truths of the Gospel. We give here, by way of illustration, two or three cases recorded by Dr. Vartan, in letters recently received from him.

Abdil Bazak, a Moslem from Genin, was admitted for cataract in both eyes. The operation was quite successful, and he left the hospital at the end of seventeen days with excellent sight, and in good spirits. This man for several years had been deprived not only of the pleasure of enjoying the objects around him, but likewise of the means of gaining a livelihood for himself and his large family. He had spent much time and money in procuring many kinds of eye-salve, and in trying many other cures, but all to no purpose. At last, a friend recommended him to go to the medical mission at Nazareth, and should he get no benefit there, then to give up all hope of recovery. He came, and the Lord blessed the operation. During his stay in the hospital, he repeatedly heard the story of Paul's journey to Damascus, and had the truths of the Gospel faithfully pressed upon his attention ; and although at first he was especially impressed with the blessing of restored vision, still, by the power of the Divine Spirit, the truth found an entrance into his heart, and his inner eye was opened to see his need of a Saviour. The last day he was in the hospital he said : " I did not come to Nazareth with a purpose like that of Paul when he went to Damascus, nor can I be the means of promoting, as he did, the fame of Jesus of Nazareth; but this I can say, I will love Him, and speak good of His name, all the days of my life."

Another case is also that of a Mohammedan youth, on whom Dr. Vartan performed the operation of lithotomy, and removed a large calculus. He has also, by the blessing of God, made a good recovery. His sufferings were excruciating, but after the operation he felt as if he had come to a new state of life, and his gratitude knew no bounds. He listened with joy to the " old, old story," and the name of Jesus became to him sweeter than anything he had ever heard of before. On leaving he went to the doctor, and presenting him with a gold Napoleon, said, " This is all I possess, and it is the sum of many many farthings earned by very hard labour, and for a long time I have had it sewn into my dress to preserve it against a time of need ; it is, therefore, not only all the money I possess, but it is what I have long cherished as a valued treasure : I wish you to take it to help you to do the work of Jesus, the Good Physician." " Had I not," writes Dr. Vartan, " had great need of such help for the work here, and had I not thought that it was good to allow him to make his offering of gratitude of what he held dear, I would not have accepted the poor man's only coin ; I accepted his gift, however, in the hope that, with his restored health, the Lord will enable him to earn many more, and at the same time keep him from setting his affection too much on earthly things. He has learned about the true Friend that sticketh closer than a brother, and may he by grace be enabled to keep close to Him."

One of the old Mohammedan chiefs living in the neighbourhood, who used to sneer at the mission, and do his utmost among his co-religionists to excite prejudice against it, at last came to acknowledge openly that the medical mission was "a most blessed institution." The circumstance which led to his change of views was as follows. His wife, whom he greatly loved, fell seriously ill. The native doctors tried every thing they could think of for her relief; one remedy after another was tried, but the sufferings of the poor patient were only aggravated. His heart was touched at last, and, setting his prejudices aside, he went to Dr. Vartan, and implored him to visit his wife. The doctor went, and found the poor woman in great agony from a large abscess in the left renal region. He inserted a trocar, and drew off a large quantity of pus; the relief experienced was almost instantaneous, and a complete cure was soon effected. This wrought such a change, that the chief went to the doctor and confessed his sorrow for having dissuaded many sufferers from coming to the dispensary, that they might escape hearing what he thought was blasphemy; but, he added, " henceforth I shall confide in, and declare the power of Him who guided you in the successful treatment of my wife." We trust his confidence, by Divine grace, may grow to a belief for his own salvation, and that of his household.

Another interesting case was that of a Greek, from Kheyan, who was admitted suffering from extensive ulceration of the leg. He remained in hospital for a long time, owing to the tedious nature of the disease; but his long residence proved a blessing, not only to him, but also to several of his fellow-sufferers. He learned much of the love of the Saviour of which he previously knew nothing; and having tasted for himself that the Lord is gracious, he ceased not to tell others of the merciful love of his Redeemer. A spirit of inquiry was thus awakened among the patients, and several were so much distressed on account of their sins, that the story of the cross was eagerly listened to. During the hours for prayer, as well as at the times set apart for interrogatory teaching, each patient seemed as if he wished to be the foremost of all in receiving instruction.

"At both morning and evening prayers," writes the

doctor, " all who are able to leave their beds, sit in a circle round me, while a portion of Scripture is read and explained in a way they can understand. In offering up prayer, Moslem and Christian kneel side by side, and ask from the Lord Jesus, for himself and herself, whatever may be needful for soul and body. In the evening, worship is conducted more like a Bible class, and whilst the domestics are always interrogated, occasionally some of the patients are questioned; and in the morning a text is given to be committed to memory by all before the time for evening prayers. They are thus occupied thinking and talking about the text, and at evening worship each patient is asked to repeat it; in this way it is hoped that every patient will leave the hospital with a good store of scriptural knowledge. The patients thoroughly enjoy their morning and evening gatherings. One evening," writes the doctor, "I asked one of the patients—and a more obstinate Mohammedan I had scarcely ever met—if he thought there was anything objectionable in our religious exercises. He said he liked them very much, and told me that till he came to the hospital he thought that he, and those only who believed and acted like himself, could please God; but now he had discovered that what he had formerly boasted of must be counted hypocrisy in God's sight. This man had a cancerous eye, which I extirpated successfully. Our morning and evening services have, I observe, a very beneficial effect upon all, even upon the most ignorant and unruly. When I make my rounds afterwards, I generally find the patients bright and cheerful, however much inclined to despondency before, and this of itself helps to promote recovery from illness; but a far more important consideration is the fact that, through Divine grace, not a few of the patients are led to see their sinful and lost state, and to seek the Saviour."

In visiting patients at their own homes, and in itinerating tours among the surrounding towns and villages, Dr. Vartan is everywhere gladly welcomed. In one of his rather extensive tours, he visited Sebastieh, Nablous, Jaffa, Ramleh, Jericho, Salt (Ramoth Gilead), Ammon, Jerash, and Gadara, and in each of these places the people soon discovered that he was a Hakim, and came to him in crowds, bringing to him their sick, or asking him to visit them at their homes. In treating their bodily infirmities he had most favourable opportunities of telling them of their souls' disease, and directing them to the Great Physician. The people were everywhere very attentive and grateful. At Salt, where the Church Missionary Society has a station, the people at first supposed that he had come with the intention of making a considerable stay, and rejoiced greatly, but when they heard that he must pass on, they were loud in their expressions of sorrow. They all, with one voice, begged him to inform his Society of their urgent need of a missionary physician, who might do so much good to the souls and bodies of the many sufferers, who die the

double death for want of such help. While there, sick
and suffering ones kept him busily engaged from morning
till night. Among the stupendous ruins of Ammon,
Jerash, and Gadara, he was welcomed by the wild Bedouins, who often molest and rob the ordinary traveller,
even in spite of his large escort. The medical missionary
is thus a participant in the joyful surprise of the seventy
on their return to their Lord (Luke x. 17).

The late Rev. W. Lindsay Alexander, D.D., in reference to what he had seen of Dr. Vartan's work a few
years ago when visiting Palestine, says : ‘‘There were
patients in his hospital at the time of my visit, not only
from the immediate neighbourhood, but even beyond
the Jordan his fame as a physician had extended, and
from thence people had brought their sick friends to be
placed under his care. I rode out with him one morning
when he was going on a professional tour—partly to see
the country and the village which he was going to visit,
Cana of Galilee, and partly to observe his manner of
work amongst the people ; and wherever he went, I
observed with pleasure the great esteem and respect in
which he was held, and the perfect confidence they
exercised in him. I was, indeed, very much impressed
with all that I saw in favour of Dr. Vartan and the work
in which he is engaged.”

One more testimony regarding the success of Dr.
Vartan's professional work. It was kindly written by
Dr. Robert Lewins, Staff Surgeon-Major, to one of the

directors of the Edinburgh Medical Missionary Society : " During a recent visit to Palestine," Dr. Lewins writes, " I had ample opportunity of witnessing the character of the duties performed by the medical missionary there, and was much impressed by their valuable nature. I was particularly struck with the success of Dr. Vartan in operative surgery—sixty cases of amputation (major) having been performed, without a single casualty—a result, so far as I am aware, unprecedented elsewhere, and which induced me to recommend Dr. Vartan to publish a detailed statement of his practice and experience in Syria, as a *desideratum* in the statistics of medical science."

We leave these facts and testimonies, which might be multiplied indefinitely, to produce their own impression. When we remember the natural aversion of the human heart to the Gospel—the prejudice, ignorance, and superstition, and the bitter enmity to the truth which characterize Mohammedanism and every other false system ; when we have such abundant evidence that, by the skilful practice of the healing art, deeply rooted prejudices are overcome, hard hearts subdued, and ready access gained to communities and homes where, as ambassadors for Christ, we desire to make known the Gospel message; and when, above all, we remember that our Divine Lord and Master Himself sanctified the medical missionary method by His own example and precept, surely no argument is needed to enforce the claims of medical missions ; yea, it is necessary rather to enforce the all-important truth, that although the medical mission principle bears the stamp of Divine approval, and commends itself to human intelligence as eminently adapted for the object in view, still that principle has no virtue in itself. In the accomplishment of His great and glorious purposes of mercy, God condescends to employ human instrumentality, but "neither is he that planteth anything, nor he that watereth, but God that giveth the increase." The agency we employ may to all human appearance be perfect, but, without the energizing influence of God's Holy Spirit, it is nothing more than a splendid machine without the motive power. The Gospel is the Divinely appointed, and only means, for the world's regeneration ; it, and it alone, under the influence of the Spirit, can turn men from darkness to light, from the power of Satan unto God; and in pleading for the more general employment of medical missions, all we here contend for is, that through medicine and surgery we gain a readier access to the homes and hearts of those whom we desire to reach with the Gospel message.

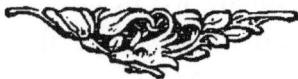

# THE VALUE OF MEDICAL MISSIONS AS A DIRECT EVANGELISTIC AGENCY.

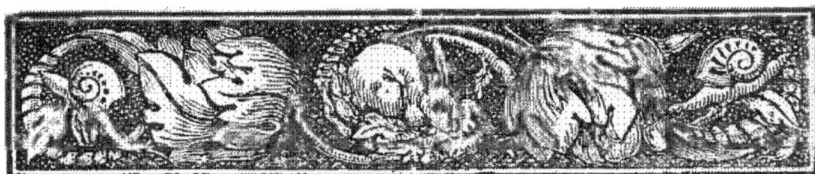

# CHAPTER IV.

### The value of Medical Missions, as a direct Evangelistic Agency, illustrated by their results in India.

FACTS and testimonies to the value of medical missions, such as have been adduced, are in themselves sufficient evidence that this department of service is no mere experiment. In many of our mission fields abroad, mission hospitals and dispensaries are now in active operation; and where they are most numerous, as in China, there their value and importance as auxiliaries to missionary effort are most gratefully acknowledged—indeed, considered by many as indispensable to the success of the work. Our missionary societies, with certain exceptions, are yet slow to recognize the medical mission as an ordinary method of missionary work, and seem disposed to minimize its employment as much as possible; and even when established, the support it receives from home is not as a rule either so hearty or so liberal as it ought to be; too often, indeed, the medical missionary has not only to do the work, but likewise to find the means for carrying it on.

This lukewarmness, or rather want of appreciation of this agency, on the part of some of our missionary societies, arises in great measure, we believe, from the erroneous impression that the practical operations of a medical mission are not so directly evangelistic as the ordinary stereotyped methods. If this can be truthfully said of any medical mission, we feel sure that, on inquiry into all the circumstances, it will be found that its usefulness as an evangelistic agency is crippled, simply because, to the bitter regret of the missionary, his professional duties are so overwhelming that he cannot possibly attempt to do more. If sufficient help were forthcoming to enable him to train and to employ native assistants—if he were relieved from the necessity of devoting so much of his time to the raising of means for the support of his mission—in short, if our missionary societies were to deal as generously with the medical mission as with the other departments of work, there would be less need to complain of the medical missionary ever allowing professional work to engross his time and attention at the expense of the evangelistic. The fault is not in the agency, nor, with very rare exceptions, in the agent, but in the exceedingly limited resources placed at his disposal to enable him to carry on his work.

We must state, however, that in our extensive and
intimate acquaintance with medical missions in all parts
of the world, we are unable to point to one which is not
a powerful influence for good, or which, viewed from an
evangelistic point of view, is not a most successful
auxiliary to missionary work. In the previous chapter,
we have entered somewhat minutely into details, especially
in the reference made to Dr. Vartan's success at Nazareth,
and have given illustrations of the evangelistic value of a
medical mission hospital and dispensary, as well as of the
special facilities afforded, in visits to patients at their own
homes, and in more or less extended medico-evangelistic
tours. Moreover, in defining the position and *status* of the
medical missionary, we have insisted upon the recognition
of his claim as an evangelist, and that, as such, he be sent
forth by the Church. It is to this feature of his mission
that we now wish especially to direct attention. All that
we have said in support of medical missions may be
accepted as scriptural, and may receive the hearty
sympathy and approval of the friends of missions, but still
their claims as a direct evangelistic agency must be
clearly shown, and convincingly apprehended, before the
enterprise for which we plead can take its proper place
in the *entourage* of missions, or be cordially and
generously supported. We shall therefore proceed to
illustrate the practical operations of medical missions, as a
direct and successful evangelistic agency in the foreign
field ; not only, as already shown, in pioneering the way,

in overcoming prejudice, and in gaining access for the Gospel messenger, but still further, that this agency is itself a method, signally owned and blessed, in winning souls to the Saviour, and in thus extending the kingdom of Christ in distant lands.

As bearing on this point, we shall begin with a few reminiscences of our own experience in Travancore.   In all the operations of the medical mission, as carried on from day to day—in the work of the hospital, the home station dispensary, the branch dispensaries and hospitals ; in visiting the sick, in and around Neyoor, and in the surrounding towns and villages ; in the training of native students as medical evangelists, and in our itinerating tours—the evangelistic element had always a prominence given to it which could not fail, with the Divine blessing, to produce a deep impression, and which we thankfully acknowledge was fruitful in spiritual results. All the students and servants of the institutions were, as far as we could judge, earnest and true-hearted Christians, and every department of the work was conducted in a prayerful, hopeful spirit.   From sixty to a hundred patients and their friends, many of them coming from a great distance, daily assembled in the waiting-room in the early morning, when the Word of God was read and expounded, and prayer offered ; and it was indeed a wonderful and interesting sight to see there, under the same roof, men and women of all castes and creéds, listening attentively to the Gospel message, and then, in outward form at least, humbly kneeling before the Majesty of heaven. After this service, while the patients were being examined and prescribed for, the native ordained evangelist, in connection with the medical mission, was occupied in the waiting-room in ministering to sin-sick souls, distributing tracts to all who could read, or reading and explaining them to such as could not, thus dealing personally with the ignorant and deluded worshippers of idols; and, moreover, as time and opportunity permitted, seeking them out at their homes, he renewed his efforts for their spiritual good. In the hospital, the same kindly interest was shown, and the same influences brought to bear upon the patients, only in much more hopeful circumstances. There were many large heathen towns and villages in which not a single Christian could be found, and where the missionary's voice was seldom, if ever, heard; into these we gained a welcome access, and while visiting the sick, enjoyed most favourable opportunities of preaching the Gospel, not only to our patients, but also to the crowds which on such occasions eagerly thronged around us.

We can conceive of no more hopeful or inviting field for evangelistic effort than that of a well-equipped medical mission, such as the one we were privileged to superintend in Travancore. Details of one or two cases will best illustrate the nature of the work, and the success which attended it. A man, belonging to the carpenter caste, accidentally inflicted a severe wound upon his right foot, splitting it up fully two inches through its entire thickness. We were absent at the time the patient was brought to the hospital, but our native assistant attended to the case, ligatured the bleeding arteries, and stitched up the wound. On our return, everything seemed to be going on so favourably that we refrained from removing the bandages, and the case was given in charge to one of the students. The wound gradually healed, and, after six weeks' residence in the hospital, he was dismissed cured. This patient, when he was admitted, knew absolutely nothing of the way of salvation;—before he left, he had a clear, and, we had every reason to believe, a saving knowledge of the truth. He expressed a strong desire for baptism before returning to his heathen home, but we thought it wise to delay for a time. He stood firm, however, against the efforts of relatives and friends to induce him to retract his new-found faith, and three months after he left the hospital he was baptized; soon after, his wife began to accompany him to religious service in the chapel, became interested in Divine things, and within a year she too was baptized.

A woman belonging to a respectable family, living in a town about twelve miles from Neyoor, was brought to the hospital, suffering from very extensive scrofulous ulceration of the leg, for which there was no alternative but amputation. The leg was amputated at the lower third of the thigh, and the wound healed so rapidly and satisfactorily, that three weeks from the day of operation,

she was able to be limping about in the verandah of the
hospital, and in five weeks from the day of admission
she was permitted to return home. Her husband and
sister were allowed to remain with her during her residence in the hospital. They were all bigoted Roman
Catholics when admitted, but the instruction they received, while inmates of the hospital, was so blessed to
them, that before they left, they renounced the false
system which they had embraced, and after a six months'
probation, they were received into the fellowship of the
Church.

Another interesting case was that of an out-door
patient, a man of much influence, and having many, both
old and young, in his employment. He was seized with
a severe attack of rheumatic fever, and being too ill to be
removed to the hospital, which was fully eight miles
distant, we visited him at his own home, and every
second day for some time after, and left a student to
attend upon him. Though he was dangerously ill, and
his case considered hopeless by his native physician and
friends, the Lord blessed the means used for his recovery, and at the same time subdued his heart, and
induced him, his wife, and several of his friends, to lend
a willing ear to the truths of the Gospel. He was soon
out of danger, and, with the exception of a stiff knee-
joint—which, however, in course of time yielded to treatment—he made a slow but good recovery, and loud were
the expressions of gratitude bestowed upon us, both by

the patient and his friends.    More pleasing than all,
however, was a message received from the patient, a few
days after we had ceased attendance upon him, asking
us, on a certain day, to come to his house along with our
assistants, in order to receive from him his devil orna-
ments, cloths, and clubs, and to demolish for him a
devil-temple (which he had built on his property only a
few months before), as he no longer had any confidence
in his idols, and had resolved, along with his wife and
several of his relatives, to join the Christians.    We gladly
accepted the invitation, and on the afternoon of the
day appointed went to our patient's house, where we met
with a most cordial reception.    A goodly congregation
having gathered within the court, we held a short service,
and then set to work with pick-axes, hatchets, and spades,
and for some time we all worked like navvies, till the
devil-temple was levelled to the ground.    Many poor,
superstitious heathen stood round us, trembling with fear,
and prophesying all kinds of evil ; the patient's wife, too,
was very nervous, and fearful that some dreadful calamity
would that very night befall them ; but her husband was
very bold, and, while watching our work, he denounced
the foolishness and vanity of his previous confidences, and
expressed, almost in the language of Joshua of old, his
determination that henceforth, " As for me and my house,
we will serve the Lord."    Having finished our icono-
clastic work outside, we adjourned to the house, where
we again had a short service, and after resting for a little,

were regaled with a sumptuous feast of curry and rice, milk, plantains, sweetmeats, &c.  Having arranged that one of our dressers should remain with the family all night, in order to comfort and encourage them, we returned to Neyoor, carrying with us the visible signs of that day's victory over the devil in one of his own strongholds.  After a few months' probation, the whole family were baptized, and it is gratifying to be able to add, that through this man's influence, and by his faithful efforts, a large number of the villagers have been led to forsake their heathen worship, and to attend regularly on the means of grace.

We give these cases, not as special and extraordinary instances, but as among many, equally interesting, occurring within a period of two months, and as examples of what we daily prayed for, and expected, as the outcome of the work.

The experience of our late lamented successor, Dr. Thomson, as recorded in his letters and annual reports, was not less encouraging.  Year by year, as the work extended, its influence as an aggressive missionary agency, became more and more evident and powerful. Branch dispensaries were multiplied, and each of these, in the locality where it was established, became a new centre of spiritual as well as of bodily healing.  As illustrative of this, we give a brief extract or two from recent reports of the work of the native medical evangelists in charge of branch dispensaries :—

"'The labours of the medical evangelist at Santha-puram," writes Dr. Thomson, "have been much blessed. The people have great confidence in him; some have been known to sell their brass vessels, to enable them to come and stay at the little hospital under his charge. The number of cases treated by him during the year is 3,609.   During the same period, sixty-six of his patients have been led, through God's blessing upon his faithful, zealous efforts, to forsake idol worship, and have put themselves under regular Christian instruction.   On the 24th of June twenty-four of these were baptized.'"

Referring to one of his cases, the dresser writes: " Sollamutto, a religious mendicant, came to the Santha-puram dispensary, some time ago, suffering from paralysis. During the time he was an in-patient, he heard the story of the cross, and became a changed man.   A proof that he is not actuated by any sinister motive, is the fact that he handed over to me his *uthiracham* (necklace of beads used by religious devotees), a small ratan, two copper rings given to him by Muttu-Kutty, and a red cloth, the means by which the mendicant gains his livelihood.   One day, being deeply convinced of his sinfulness and need of his Saviour, he said to me, ' I am near the grave ; I feel my time here is very short, and I wish to be baptized this Sunday.'   In accordance with his request, the pastor visited him, and finding that he took Jesus at His word, and simply trusted Him, he gladly baptized him on the 12th of October.   His words on that occasion were very expressive, and his face, beaming with joy, showed that he was not exaggerating what he felt in his heart. He said, 'I thank God I came to the knowledge of Jesus Christ in the dispensary. My new faith gives me true happiness. Jesus has cleansed me, and lives now in my heart, so that, day by day, I am drawn nearer and nearer to Him.' He has great joy in attending the daily dispensary services. I have special cause to remember this case, as it is the first-fruit of my feeble effort since the lamented death of my beloved master, Dr. T. S. Thomson." (Dr. Thomson died on the 31st of July, 1884.)

With reference to the work of another branch dispensary, Dr. Thomson writes : "No month goes past without reports of some being influenced to decide for Christ, or of having put themselves under Christian instruction. One dresser has made an analysis of such cases, in connection with his branch dispensary for the year, with the following results : Total number of patients who have embraced Christianity, eighty-one; of these seventy-five are regular until now in attendance at chapel, and twenty-seven have been examined and found suitable for baptism. Their names are all given, with the congregations they attend."

"Last year," writes a dresser in charge of another branch dispensary, "in one village (Peruvilei) twenty persons were baptized under the efforts of the medical mission, and there are others who, though not yet bap-

tized, are steadfast in their faith ; and on the 30th of
January, at another village in the same district, eighteen
of my former patients were baptized by the Rev. William
Lee.   As battles won," he adds, "encourage soldiers, so
to every one who is a soldier in the army of Jesus,
victories such as these are a source of great encouragement."

The native medical evangelists have all been trained,
either by the late Dr. Thomson, or by ourselves, at the
Neyoor Mission Hospital, and, from personal observation,
we can testify to their skill and success in the treatment
of disease, as well as to their faithfulness and zeal as
evangelists.   The influence they have among their fellow-
countrymen is very great, and they have access where
the ordinary native agent dare not approach.   Their
salary is not more than fifteen rupees—equal to about
thirty shillings—a month ; and to their credit be it known,
that several of them have again and again refused salaries
double or treble what they receive as agents of the
mission, rather than relinquish direct mission work.

From the south of India we pass to the extreme north,
and take a glimpse of medical mission work in Kashmir.
Here, to quote again the words of the late Lord Bishop
of Calcutta, we find the medical missionary "knocking at
the one door which may, through God's help, be opened
for the truth to enter in."   The Church Missionary
Society made an effort to introduce Christianity into
Kashmir in 1854, but the violent opposition the mis-

sionaries then encountered obliged them at once to withdraw, and it was not till 1862 that the attempt was renewed. In the autumn of that year, two missionaries visited the valley, but were again obliged to retire. Another effort was made in the following year, but the time had not yet come for the establishment of a Christian mission. In 1865, in circumstances apparently as unfavourable, a medical mission for Kashmir was again proposed. Dr. Elmslie was sent out, and, writing from Srinagar, the capital of Kashmir, very soon after his arrival, he says : " So bitter had been the opposition of the native authorities to the praiseworthy efforts of Messrs. Smith and Clark, ordained missionaries of the Church Missionary Society, on two previous occasions, that, on my arrival, I fully expected to meet with similar treatment, but I was most agreeably disappointed. With one exception, the people heard us gladly, and not the people only, but the public functionaries also." Writing about his work the following year, Dr. Elmslie says : " The religious exercises of the dispensary were conducted in the same manner as last year. On all occasions, without a single exception, the behaviour of the people was quiet and attentive. In our addresses seldom was there any express reference made to the absurdities of Hinduism, or to the errors of the religion of the false prophet; we deem such references better fitted for the solitary interview than for the crowded assembly. We wish our hearers to know what Christianity is—to look at it with their mind's eye

calmly and dispassionately; and, if we know anything of
the workings of the human mind, we believe that one of
the main ways of effecting this is not unnecessarily to
rouse the prejudices of your heathen listeners.    The
surpassing reasonableness and excellency of the Christian
religion should be the chief theme of the preacher to a
heathen audience, leaving them to institute a comparison
between their own corrupt and false religion and that of
Jesus Christ.

"We have here a good deal fitted to discourage us,
but the thought that during the past six months more
than three thousand sufferers from serious maladies have
been either wholly cured, or have had their pains alleviated—the thought that the wondrous story of God's
marvellous love to a sin-ruined world, in the stupendous
gift of His own dear Son, has become extensively known
among this people so prejudiced and exclusive—and the
absolute certainty of the final triumph of the Gospel, here
and throughout the world, should nerve and encourage
us to advance joyfully and hopefully in our Divine
Master's great and good work."

Through these many years, the medical mission has
been steadily carried on.    Under Dr. Elmslie the dispensary won a reputation throughout the whole valley.
After his death the work was carried on by different
missionaries.    Dr. Maxwell, the immediate successor of
Dr. Elmslie, was sent out in 1874, and by his influence
with the Maharajah a hospital was erected.    Under the

pressure of work his health broke down, and he was obliged to return home. During the interval previous to Dr. Downes' arrival, the work was carried on by the Rev. T. Wade and a native doctor. After six years of hard but successful work, Dr. Downes has also been compelled by ill-health to retire, and now Dr. Neve carries on the work. "The fame of the hospital," writes Dr. Neve, "has reached into remote valleys, crossed snowy passes to Ladák and Skardo, and even penetrated with merchant caravans into Khotan and Yarkand. As its fame has spread, so has its work increased. Any one who looked through the out-patient room on a crowded summer day would not quickly forget the sight of the hundreds of sick. Here the dark faces of the natives from the plains contrast with the fair Kashmiris, and the ruddy-complexioned Yarkundi; here are the fierce features of the Afghan, there the stalwart form of the Sikh, with many another strange nationality. Seven or eight different dialects or languages may be heard. Varying yet more than race and language would be the diseases and appearance of the sufferers. The child leads in his blind father, the mother carries her lame daughter, friends bring, on a light bedstead, the palsied man. The repulsive features of the leper, the disfigured countenances and ulcerated limbs of many, would inspire with horror, their wretched garments and wasted forms would fill with pity, and the painfully numerous proofs of dirty habits and vicious tastes would excite disgust.

" When gathered together, a hymn is sung, and afterwards a short address is given.  Avoiding any approach
to controversy, they are told of the God of love, and of
redemption : of Him who, as man, experienced the toils
and trials of manhood, sounded the depths of poverty,
and bore the strokes of persecution ; of Him who comforted the sorrow-stricken, healed the sick, taught the
ignorant, loved all men, died for all men, and rose again,
the first-fruits of them that sleep, now sitting at the right
hand of the Eternal Father, offering salvation to all who
call upon His name.

" To all this, whether Hindu, Buddhist, or Mohammedan, they listen with interest, and in the petitions of
the closing prayer many audibly join.  Now begins the
consulting and dispensing.  The doctor registers the
name, examines the patient, and writes the prescription,
while two compounders are at work dispensing ; one man
shows the patients in, one by one ; two more are engaged
dressing, while the native hospital assistant stands by
to look after them, performing any minor operations
or examining more carefully any special case.   So the
patients are passed through, receiving their medicines as
they go—the serious cases receiving an admission ticket
into the hospital.   At last, after several hours' work, and
after a glance through the wards, the day's work is over.
Two days a week are reserved for operations, and for a
closer inspection of the wards."

The extent of the work is great, and the number of

patients very large. It reached its maximum in 1881, when 30,000 visits were registered. Last year 8000 new cases were seen, and these paid 24,000 visits. Over 1200 operations were performed, and 1000 patients were received into the wards. These figures give some idea of the amount of work performed; but they do not include all, for many hundreds were seen by Dr. Downes at Gulmarg, and Dr. Neve and his assistant saw hundreds more while itinerating in the district. During the past six years upwards of 130,000 visits have been received, and reckoning from the commencement of the work, twenty years ago, more than twice that number.

Referring to the opportunities afforded by the Medical Mission for evangelistic work in Kashmir, the Rev. J. Hinton Knowles, Dr. Neve's colleague, writes : " If anything will help to bring about, under the Heavenly blessing, the fulfilment of these blessed words, ' At the name of Jesus every knee shall bow, of things in heaven and things on earth,' and 'every tongue shall confess that He is Christ, to the glory of God the Father,' I believe it is this noble, grand, Gospel Medical Mission. . . . Some may ask, ' What are the results of this apparently great and holy work ? How many Christians are being gathered in ?' Now and again, one and another have stepped out of the ranks of a false religion, and are now walking in the new and living way. We are striving, praying, and expecting that many will soon follow. There are several who, after the delivery of the addresses and

the distribution of the medicines, have come to inquire
more of 'these strange things brought to their ears.' The
other morning five men came all at one time. Who can
measure the blessing attending such work! Sometimes
there are as many as two hundred patients and others
present. They have come from different parts—from
over yonder snow-capped mountains, looking so near,
and yet so far off; from yonder distant village several
have come who have perhaps no other reason for visiting
Srinagar than to get advice and medicine, and to them,
and to all, the Gospel is faithfully preached. Suppose
only fifty thus hear it every day. Then that probably
means that the substance of the address is known before
nightfall to about two hundred; for, in the ordinary
routine of their life, the native has so little transpiring of
a newsful character, that he or she will be certain to
remember much of the Word spoken, and to tell it to
their families and in their *hujras* on their return. We
hear from time to time of the Gospel being thus carried
to others, with saving power: Were it not for the
Medical Mission, such splendid opportunities as we now
enjoy for preaching in the city bazaar here is practically
impossible."

One more glimpse before we turn from Kashmir.
"Itineration," writes Dr. Neve, "is a very interesting
feature of our work. Throughout the past year, preaching and the healing art have, hand in hand, visited many
of the smaller towns in the district. In the Wizier Gar-

den at Islamabad, under the chenar groves at Pampoor, by the broad placid river at Sopir, in the visitors' bungalow at Baramulla, the busy portal of the 'Happy Valley,' in the stately gardens at Vernag and Atchibal, by the sacred tank at Bâwun, below the great mosque at Eishmakâm, among the walnut trees and orchards of sequestered mountain villages, have the message of Divine love and the ministry of healing been brought to the sinful and the sick. Perhaps the most noteworthy of all these scenes was at Bâwun—most sacred of tanks, most beautiful of camps—with its smooth, grassy terrace, watered by swift-flowing canals, and canopied by the massy foliage of stately plane trees. In such a gem of natural loveliness, disease should cease to be ; but here hundreds have day by day surrounded my tent. By the limpid flashing water of the tank, pundit and fakir, Mohammedan official and peasant, have listened to the story of the 'Fountain opened for sin'—not the holy Ganges, nor this pure spring, but the life-blood of the God-man, Christ Jesus."

In Rajpootana, four European medical missionaries are at work in connection with the United Presbyterian Church. Into Jeypore, the capital, the Gospel first gained an entrance through medical missions, and in the province, since then, their value, as an evangelistic method, has been abundantly proved, and the United Presbyterian Church has wisely multiplied their number. We must allow one of the medical missionaries in Rajpootana to speak for

all. Dr. Somerville, of Beawr, thus writes : " To com-
municate, with healing for the various diseases brought to
us for treatment, a knowledge of the one true God, and
of Jesus Christ whom He hath sent, is the method and
aim of the work—not, as some injuriously represent, with
the object of forcibly, or cowardly, taking advantage of
our patients' weakness, or incapacity for thought or intelligent decision, but to show that our religion is one of
love and mercy, and that we desire to carry out the injunction of our Master, 'to preach the kingdom of God,
and to heal the sick.' In the mission dispensary all are
free to come and go, and the Gospel is shown to be a
thing, not of compulsion, but of persuasion, to the end
that sinful men may see, and accept, a Saviour from sin
in Jesus Christ. The Word has certainly been listened
to with great attention, and gained an entrance into the
understanding of many, and some have had their hearts
touched by the story of redeeming love. If it be true of
any department of Christian work, it is emphatically true
of the work of the medical missionary, that much of its
result, and even of its operation, must remain unseen and
unnoted. Even to appreciate some of its outward
aspects, one must accompany the missionary physician,
morning by morning, to the dispensary—must see the
bent and festering limbs made straight, vision restored
to the sightless eyes, pain relieved by a stroke of the
knife, and, withal, rebuke and exhortation administered
to such as are suffering from former ill-doing, and the

Word of Life read and explained to all. He must also accompany him—it may be after his dispensary work is over in the morning, it may be at any hour of the day or night—into the streets and lanes of the town, to the house of some one too ill to come to the dispensary, or to wait till the dispensary hour, and see relief administered to husband, or wife, or child, as the physician knows how ; and while waiting, or after what may be necessary has been done, to hear the message again delivered, and the attention of patient and bystander directed to things eternal. He must go with the missionary to the neighbouring or more distant village in the early morning, or from village to village on his longer itineracy, and see there the crowd collected round the village *hathai*, and observe the remedy supplied from the medicine chest for bodily ailment, and note how the sinful soul is directed to the Heavenly Physician for spiritual healing ;—all this, and much more he must do, ere a just conception can be formed of the value of the medical missionary's work. In all these ways, in common with my medical missionary brethren, I have been engaged during the past year, as in former years, preaching the Gospel and healing the sick, in the dispensary, in the house, in the lane, by the wayside, in the village, or wherever the opportunity offered. We have made a large number of visits in the bazaar, to those who were either too weak to come to the hospital, or whose social customs forbid their appearing in public ; and it is encouraging to state that, in some instances, the way has thus been opened up for more extended usefulness."

We wish we could take a glimpse of the other medical missions established by the United Presbyterian Church in Rajpootana ; but this is unnecessary, as the testimony of Dr. Husband, Dr. Shepherd, and Dr. Clark, would, in effect, be similar to that of Dr. Somerville. They each make their medical work, not the chief end, but a means to the higher end—namely, that of directing their patients, diseased by sin, to the Divine and only Physician of souls. With the experience of medical mission work which the United Presbyterian Mission Board has had in India, China, and elsewhere, it is gratifying to be able to add the following testimony from the late Rev. Dr. McGill, late Foreign Mission Secretary of that Board, to the value of this agency as a method of missionary work : "The experience of our Mission Board with reference to medical missions, which extends not only to Old Calabar and Rajpootana, but also to China, has amply verified the principles on which they have been founded. It is the settled conviction of those best acquainted with the subject, that this form of agency is stamped with the approbation of that Great Teacher, who 'went about all Galilee, teaching in their synagogues, and healing all manner of sickness and all manner of disease among the people.' From the month of September, 1855, when our first medical missionary, Dr. Hewan, went to Calabar, until the present hour, the results of our medical missions have amply vindicated their institution."

We might refer at length to the medical missions of the Church Missionary Society in the Punjab, to that of the Church of Scotland in Chumba, of the Irish Presbyterian Church in Gujerat, of the Baptist Missionary Society in Delhi, and of the Free Church of Scotland in Pachamba and Madras, as well as to that of the American Board, in connection with their Arcot Mission, but we shall content ourselves with a brief allusion to the latter, as illustrative of the work and evangelistic opportunities of all.

The hospital and dispensary in connection with the American Arcot Mission is located at Ranipett, with a branch dispensary at Wallajapett, and the work is superintended by Dr. H. M. Scudder, one of a large family of missionaries, whose name is a household word among native Christians throughout a large district in South India. This Institution was established in 1866. At first, the people came cautiously and timidly, and usually from the lowest castes; now, all is changed, Hindus of the highest castes and Mohammedans alike avail themselves of its benefits without the shadow of a fear, the average annual attendance of out-patients being upwards of 30,000, and of in-patients about 1300.

The Gospel is preached daily at the dispensary. As the patients arrive they are seated upon benches in the large verandah of the building, and when a goodly number have gathered, a portion of Scripture is read, and the truth made known as simply and clearly as possible. The in-patients, lying in their beds in the adjoining wards, are able to hear distinctly all that is said. The branch dispensary at Wallajapett is very much appreciated, crowds resorting to it day by day, and there, as at Ranipett, precious opportunities are enjoyed of sowing the good seed in a specially prepared soil. Attendance at those services is by no means compulsory; all are invited, but if unwilling to remain they are at perfect liberty to retire. Very rarely, however, do any absent themselves; all listen attentively, and with apparent interest.

"It may be asked," writes Dr. Scudder, "whether this method of evangelization is successful. Most assuredly it is, though, perhaps, we may never know how much good is accomplished until the last great day. Many cases of conversion have occurred within the walls of the hospital, and numbers of others, who have come over to us, have affirmed that the preaching they heard on the dispensary verandah first led them to inquire after the truth. Do Christian friends—do even all missionaries—appreciate the great importance of medical missionary work? We very much fear they do not. We consider that every mission ought to have, at least, one arm medical; that is, should have an efficient medical department in connection with it. Yet how many missions are still without this agency. Surely this is a poor policy, looking at the subject even from a worldly point of view;

but, when we know that the medical missionary has a new, extensive, easily attainable, but otherwise unapproachable field—most interesting as well as hopeful—upon which he may enter almost immediately, and with scarcely an obstacle in his pathway, is it not manifest that this subject should have, as it certainly deserves to have, much more attention? God grant that the claims of medical missions may more seriously enter into the hearts and minds of His people everywhere, and arouse them to extend this special field of labour and usefulness!"

We cannot better conclude this brief reference to the evangelistic results of medical mission work in India than by the following testimony of a learned Brahmin. At the close of a lecture by Dr. Chamberlain, of the American Arcot Mission, when nearly two hundred Brahmins, farmers, artizans, officials, and students were present, the Brahmin politely asked permission to address the meeting, and then said:

"I have watched the missionaries, and seen what they are. What have they come to this country for? What tempts them to leave their parents, friends, and country, and come to this, to them, unhealthy clime? Is it for gain or profit they come? Some of us, country clerks in Government offices, receive larger salaries than they. Is it for an easy life? See how they work, and then tell me. Look at this missionary! He came here a few years ago, leaving all, and seeking only our good! He

was met with cold looks and suspicious glances, and was
shunned and maligned. He sought to talk with us of
what, he told us, was the matter of most importance in
heaven and earth, but we would not listen. He was not
discouraged ; he opened a dispensary, and we said, ' Let
the pariahs (lowest caste people) take his medicines, we
won't ;' but in the time of our sickness and distress and
fear we were glad to go to him, and he welcomed us.
We complained at first if he walked through our Brahmin
streets ; but ere long, when our wives and our daughters
were in sickness and anguish, we went and begged him
to come, even into our inner apartments—and he came,
and our wives and our daughters now smile upon us in
health ! Has he made any money by it ? Even the cost
of the medicine he has given has not been returned to
him.

"Now what is it that makes him do all this for us ?
*It is his Bible !* I have looked into it a good deal, at
one time or another, in the different languages I chance
to know ; it is just the same in all languages. The
Bible !—there is nothing to compare with it, in all our
sacred books, for goodness, and purity, and holiness, and
love, and for motives of action. Where did the English
people get all their intelligence and energy, and clever-
ness and power ? It is their Bible that gives it to them.
And now they bring it to us and say, ' That is what raised
us, take it and raise yourselves !' They do not force it
upon us, as did the Mohammedans with their Koran ;

but they bring it in love, and translate it into our languages, and lay it before us, and say, ' Look at it, read it, examine it, and see if it is not good.' Of one thing I am convinced : do what we will, oppose it as we may, it is the Christian's Bible that will, sooner or later, work the regeneration of our land."

"I could not," adds Dr. Chamberlain, "but be surprised at this testimony. Some time ago, I had attended in his zenana, his second wife, a beautiful girl, through a dangerous illness, and I knew that he was very grateful, but I was not prepared to hear him, before such an audience, give such a powerful testimony to the power and excellence of the Bible."

In view of the results of medical missionary work in India, and with testimony to its value such as we have given, are we not reminded of the words of Moses in his song of triumph ? "Their rock is not as our rock, even our enemies themselves being judges "; and were this agency more largely made use of in that "land of idols," such testimony would doubtless be more frequently heard.

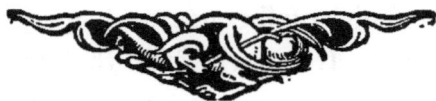

# THE VALUE OF MEDICAL MISSIONS AS A
# DIRECT EVANGELISTIC AGENCY.

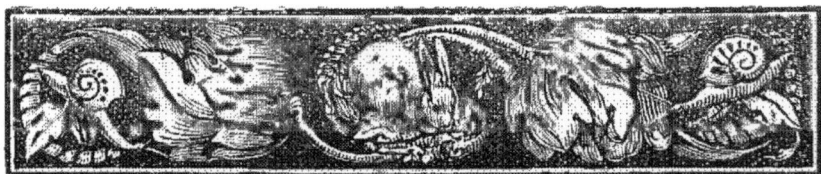

## CHAPTER V.

The value of Medical Missions as a direct Evangelistic Agency, illustrated by their results in China and elsewhere.

NOWHERE is the evangelistic value of medical missionary work better illustrated than in China. We shall now, therefore, take a glimpse at some of the mission hospitals and dispensaries in that great mission field. Our object, let it be borne in mind, in this, as in the previous chapter, is not so much to illustrate the influence of medical missions, in disarming prejudice and pioneering a way for the proclamation of the Gospel— this we have already done; our aim is rather to show how fruitful medical missions are in their direct evangelistic results—how manifestly God has blessed this agency in winning souls to the Saviour, and that from this point of view alone, medical missions have, therefore, a very strong claim upon the sympathy and support of the friends of missions.

In 1834, the Rev. Peter Parker, M.D., of the American Board of Missions, arrived in China; the first medical missionary to that great empire. His hospital in Canton soon became so popular, that patients of all ranks, and from distant parts of the country flocked to it. In 1839 Dr. Lockhart, the agent of the London Missionary Society, arrived and commenced work in Macao; towards the close of the same year, he was joined by Dr. Hobson. The operations of those pioneers of medical missionary work in China were, for a short time, interrupted by the breaking out of hostilities in 1840. When peace was restored, Dr. Lockhart went to Shanghai and Dr. Hobson to Hongkong. Excellent mission hospitals were built and furnished at both places, and both missionaries were greatly blessed in their "work of faith and labour of love."

Dr. Lockhart, speaking of the work which he was thus privileged to inaugurate, says : "In 1838 I was sent out by the London Missionary Society as their first medical missionary to China. A house was taken for a dispensary and hospital, and the people were informed that they would receive gratuitous medical attendance. They came in great numbers, so that in the course of a few weeks our house was quite full, and the street was crowded every morning with patients flocking to us for aid; and it was pleasant to see how soon, by this work of humanity, we could find a way to their affections and their hearts, and how the people who were thus relieved would dwell upon the words of the preacher. I believe the truth thus found its way to the hearts of many who, without the hospital, would never have known the glad tidings of the Gospel. Many persons came from the northern and western provinces to our hospital at Shanghai. When under treatment there, they heard the Gospel preached. Returning to their distant homes, they took with them portions of the Word of God, and various religious tracts; and thus the message of salvation found its way into large districts of country which, without this agency, we had no means of reaching. This is the great object of medical missions. We strive to win the confidence of the people—to get them around us—to open their hearts by kindness to receive the Divine Word—and thus, sowing the seed at a favourable time, bring many to know Christ, whose hearts might otherwise be prejudiced against His truth. We repeatedly heard of patients who, having been to the hospital, and having there heard the Gospel, carried with them portions of the Word of God to their native villages, and induced others of their friends to come down in order to participate in the same benefits. So the work went on, and I say it with confidence, that medical missions in China have been successful in winning an entrance for the Gospel to the hearts and consciences of the people, which no other agency could have so well effected."

About this time very valuable testimony, to the remarkable influence and success of those early medical missionary operations among the Chinese, was borne by an intelligent eye-witness, Dr. Wilson, Inspector of Naval Hospitals, who, in his work entitled " Medical Notes on China," thus refers to medical missions : "Among the most promising means now employed for reforming, or rather revolutionizing, the moral, intellectual, and social condition of the Chinese, we would rank the medical missions recently established on their shores.   In their frequent, and, from its very nature, familiar intercourse with the afflicted, the medical missionaries possess advantages, which the man who addresses himself to the understanding only canno obtain.   They have consequently more potent means of touching the heart, and turning feelings of gratitude into instruments by which they may act powerfully on the dark mind.   Though they do not directly assail the strongholds of bigotry and conceited ignorance, they trust that, through the agency of accumulated good works, which can neither excite jealousy in rulers, nor permit continued indifference among the people, so to undermine these antiquated structures, that they may ere long annihilate them, rearing in their room institutions of light and liberty; substituting for the worship of idols, adoration of the true God.

"The hospital of the medical mission at Hongkong, which is under the direction of Dr. Hobson, and which is best know to us, may be taken as a general representative of those established at other ports. There, everything which benevolence can devise, and care and skill accomplish, is done for the patients ; and thence, a large proportion of those admitted return to their native towns and hamlets, to tell their neighbours what the strangers have done for them. They have to speak only of benefits received; their cherished habits were not violently attacked ; their superstitious follies and pagan perversions were never made the subjects of ridicule or contemptuous pity, but they were led to the abandonment of these by showing them a better way, and by proving its vast superiority through its practical results. Persons who went in wasted, maimed, or blind, came out with renovated vigour and restored sight. Can the Chinese long continue to resist such teaching ? "

Since these first mission hospitals were established in China, medical missions have been intimately associated with the progress of missionary work there. There are now between forty and fifty missionary physicians, European and American, carrying on their Christ-like labours in all parts of that vast empire, and a brief reference to a few of the mission hospitals and dispensaries under their charge will serve to show how valuable they are as direct evangelistic agencies.

The Rev. Griffith John, one of the most experienced and best known missionaries in China, writing regarding the London Missionary Society's Medical Mission at

Hankow, says: "I am happy to be able to state that our hospital at Hankow is a thoroughly Christian institution. Every helper is, so far as we are able to judge, a genuine disciple of the Lord Jesus Christ, and in perfect sympathy with the higher aim of the establishment. From end to end, and from top to bottom, the atmosphere of the hospital is a purely religious one. So actively engaged are the assistants in making known the truth to the patients, that it is almost impossible for any one to spend three or four days within the building without obtaining a fair knowledge of the fundamental truths of the Gospel. I never enter the wards without feeling that the institution is a great spiritual power, and that it is destined to accomplish a mighty work for God in the centre of China."

The Hankow Mission Hospital was built in 1874, largely by funds raised among the Chinese themselves. The land was a gift to the hospital by Dr. Reid, who for many years freely gave his time to the medical work of the mission. Accommodation is provided for about forty patients, and out-patients are seen five days a week. " Every day," writes the medical missionary, " when the patients are assembled in the waiting-room, the Gospel is proclaimed to them. That they get a clear mental knowledge of the truth we know, by the intelligent answers given to the frequent questions asked in the consulting-room. Those who remain as in-patients receive daily religious instruction, and through kindness and attention to their bodily sufferings, we seek to lead them to the Great Physician, who alone can meet their spiritual wants."

"Patients come from great distances for advice and treatment, even from the provinces of Hu-nan and Kian-si. From Mien-Yaang alone, though over a hundred miles distant, we have had twenty-three in-patients during the year. In this way, the Gospel reaches many who would never probably have come under its influence in any other way, for their homes have not yet been reached by missionary effort. Many take away with them a knowledge, at least, of the way of salvation, and not a few return to their homes humble disciples of the Lord Jesus."

Among many most interesting cases, the medical missionary tells us of a father, a small farmer, who brought his two daughters, aged thirteen and sixteen, to the hospital, suffering from cataract of both eyes and totally blind. Both girls were operated upon and returned home with their sight restored. While in the hospital they received daily Christian instruction, and, by and by, both expressed an earnest desire to confess Christ. After a few weeks' probation, having given satisfactory evidence of a real change of heart, they were baptized. Three months after leaving the hospital, they again appeared with a number of sick and maimed neighbours, their mother being one of the party. She had been blind from cataract for upwards of twenty years, and was now forty years old. She had not come to Hankow, she said, to be cured, for after so many years' blindness she could never expect to be able to see, but she had come to receive Christian instruction ; her daughters had told her much about the Gospel, and she was anxious now for urther knowledge. Her case, happily, was not con-sidered hopeless ; both eyes were successfully operated upon, and her sight was restored. While in the hospital both she and her husband were led to know Jesus as their Saviour, were baptized the Sunday before they left, and returned to their home a Christian family.

The largest medical mission in China is that in con-nection with the English Presbyterian Church at Swatow, which was commenced in 1863 by Dr. Gauld, in a Chinese house fitted up to accommodate a few in-patients. In 1867 a new hospital was built, with accommodation for from fifty to sixty patients, with a separate house in another part of the town used exclusively as a leper hospital. Since then the work has expanded with a steady growth, till now there is hospital accommodation for two hundred patients, and at times room has to be found for a considerably larger number. Till 1877 Dr. Gauld carried on the work single-handed ; failure of health, however, obliged him to retire from the foreign field, about two years ago, but he is now doing good service as Superintendent of the Bethnal Green Medical Mission, in connection with the Mildmay Mission. In 1877 Dr. Lyall, formerly resident physician at the Cowgate Dispensary, was sent out to assist Dr. Gauld, and he has now sole charge of the Swatow Medical Mission.

During 1883, upwards of one hundred and forty patients, men and women, gave in their names as candidates for church fellowship. For such, special classes are held, more or less regularly during the week, and on Sunday afternoons they assemble for examination on the subjects taught. Of this large number of applicants only a few were baptized, previous to their leaving the hospital, the missionaries as a rule requiring that, before receiving baptism, they should go home and show the sincerity of their profession by conducting themselves as Christians among their relatives and neighbours. Many of those who receive a blessing themselves while inmates in the hospital are very zealous and successful in bringing in others for instruction. In a recent report, Dr. Lyall gives several very interesting cases of conversion, the result of such efforts. One patient, baptized in 1881, brought his mother and younger brother, a three days' journey to Swatow, to receive Christian instruction; now both are applicants for admission into the Church. Another, baptized on the 1st of January, 1881, has influenced a number of his friends in favour of the Gospel; and his brother, who came several times to Swatow to receive teaching, has been baptized. A man from Chiahna, when under treatment towards the end of 1880, became very anxious about his soul's salvation, found peace in believing, and desired to join the Church, but his baptism was delayed in order that the sincerity of his wish might be tested. On his return to his village, his conduct was so changed as to make his old comrades and his neighbours wonder what had come over him. Formerly he had been addicted to gambling, swearing, and other evil habits, but now he was an example to all in his daily life and conversation. After a short probation he was baptized, became a most intelligent, zealous, useful Christian, and was recently elected an office-bearer of the Church at Chiah-na.

In the end of May, 1878, one of three patients baptized in the hospital was Ung-A-Che, a leper. He came from Na-than, a large village near the head of Chaw-an-basin, not long ago notorious for the piratical habits of the people. After a stay of several months in the hospital, A-Che applied for baptism, and after due examination was received into the Church. He returned to his home soon after, not cured of his leprosy, but rejoicing in Christ as his Saviour. "We heard nothing of him," writes the Rev. H. L. Mackenzie of Swatow, "until the beginning of 1882. His village is fully two and a half days' journey from here, and in a region to which none of us had ever paid a visit. Well, to our surprise and delight we heard that, through A-Che's preaching of the Gospel to his neighbours, some twenty or thirty men and women, from his own and two neighbouring villages, had turned from the worship of idols to serve the living God, and were in the habit of meeting regularly to worship Him. We sent our native assistant to inquire into this new and interesting movement, and to teach and encourage those who professed to be converts. The report he brought back was well fitted to make us very hopeful as to the reality of the work, and we looked forward to visiting the place soon. For various reasons the visit did not take place till very recently, and I wish now to tell you what Dr. Lyall and I found at Na-than when we spent a few days there. Arriving early in July, we were warmly welcomed by several of the brethren, A-Che being among them. I at once recognized the poor fellow. He is much disfigured in face and limb by the sad dreadful disease, that is slowly, but surely, bringing him down to the grave; but there was a peaceful, happy expression of face that touched me deeply, and I could but bless the Lord, for the grace given to our afflicted brother, and wonder and adore when I thought of the honour put upon him. He and the others conducted us to their meeting-place. It was an open lane, just in front of the house of one of the brethren, and with openings into it from the houses of the neighbours. They had been trying hard, for more than a year, to get a house or even a single room wherein to meet, but had failed; and so Dr. Lyall and I met with them where they regularly assembled for worship, exposed to the heat and to the cold, to a blazing sun and to heavy rains. We found a small congregation of twenty-seven souls; a few of the more prominent and decided men happened on that day

to be from home.  To shelter us from the hot sun, a few
pine branches, and one or two pieces of what looked like
old sail-cloth, had been spread over head.  The men sat
on small forms, the women squatted on straw mats spread
on the ground ; for Dr. Lyall and myself a couple of
bamboo chairs had been provided."  In this strange
place, Mr. Mackenzie and Dr. Lyall spoke to these people,
and after careful examination of those who had applied
for baptism, two men and three women were baptized.
" We were glad and thankful," Mr. Mackenzie adds, " for
what we had seen of the grace of God, and praised Him
for so wonderfully opening the way to Na-than, and that
our first visit there was so encouraging and happy."

The visits of the ladies of the mission to the female
patients in their wards have been much blessed.  The
matron of the girls' school, who was herself led to become
a Christian while a patient in the hospital many years
ago, and who has been very useful to many of her people
since, often spends an hour among the women, when free
from her school duties.  As a result of these efforts,
some very interesting conversions have taken place
among them.

At a meeting held lately in the medical mission house,
Edinburgh, the Rev. Mr. Macgregor of Amoy gave a
most interesting account of medical mission work in
China, and among other gratifying results he told of a
man from an unevangelized district of country who came,
nearly seventeen years ago, to the hospital at Amoy,

where he was cured of his disease and received daily Christian instruction. When quite recovered, he returned home and told his friends and neighbours of the kind treatment he had received, and of the Gospel of God's love which he had heard. The hearts of a few were opened, and they believed, the number increased, persecution arose, at one time so fierce that they had to flee from the village. At length they communicated with the missionaries and begged for a teacher; one was sent, and a congregation of about a hundred was gathered. Many came from a considerable distance, and a new community had to be formed further inland; the work has gone on increasing, "and to-day," said Mr. Macgregor, "there are seven congregations, each numbering from thirty to upwards of a hundred persons, all the outcome of God's blessing upon the good seed sown in that one patient's heart, while in the mission hospital."

The medical mission of the Church Missionary Society at Hangchow has been in operation for fourteen years. Dr. Galt began the work there, and for nearly eight years carried it on with much success. In 1879 he was obliged to retire from the foreign field, owing to the failure of his wife's health. In the autumn of 1881, Dr. Main was sent out as Dr. Galt's successor, and has had much success in his work. The hospital recently erected has accommodation for seventy in-patients, and includes a commodious dispensary and waiting-room for out-patients. In his report for 1884, Dr. Main thus states the result of

his experience : " Medical missions are indeed a grand
weapon in the hand of God for removing prejudice,
winning the affections of the people, and at the same
time directing their minds to Christ.   It is the privilege
of the medical missionary not only to ' heal,' but also to
' preach,' to care for the soul as well as for the body.
To do his work thoroughly, however, he must be well
supported.   He should have plenty of well-trained assistants, to relieve him of all the heavy and drudgery work of
the hospital and dispensary.   He should not be expected
to dress every ulcer, or attend to trifling or minor details.
If the medical missionary has to attend to everything
himself, he will soon find out that he must either break
down, or allow the grand side of his work to be neglected,
and thereby lose the joy of ' telling out among the
heathen the story of redeeming love.'

" With the in-patients we have a service morning and
evening, consisting of a short Gospel address, singing
and prayer.   In our visits to the wards, we trust the
patients all know that our chief desire and object is to
benefit their souls as well as their bodies.   Every Sunday
afternoon we have an interesting Bible-reading and prayer
meeting, with the assistants, pupils, servants, and Christian patients, should there be any ; we have found this
meeting a great help in our work.   In the evening we
have an open Gospel meeting, when those who desire to
do so may testify to what the Lord has done for them.
We have opened a reading-room lately, where any one

may come in and read the Scriptures, and other books and tracts that lie on the tables. Every night of the week it is open for preaching, and quite a number come in ; a few have come every night for weeks, professing to be interested in the ' doctrine.'

"On dispensary days, twice a week, out-patients assemble in the waiting-room, where, before receiving advice, they are told of the Great Physician of souls, receive tracts, &c. Short itinerating tours into the district are made from time to time ; on one of these, lately, a Buddhist priest invited me to open my medicine chest in his temple, and there, surrounded with gods of wood and clay, I examined my patients and gave them medicines, and at the same time told them of the one living and true God.

"As to results, we have every reason to thank God and take courage. The hand of the Lord has indeed been with us. The Gospel has been preached to thousands, and carried in the hand, head, or heart, to all parts of the country."

Four years ago, Dr. Christie was sent out by the United Presbyterian Church to commence medical mission work in Manchuria. Hitherto he has had to devote the greater part of his time to the study of the language, and to superintending the erection of his hospital and dispensary ; still he has had large numbers of patients coming to him, and in writing of his evangelistic work, he says, that while he regards the alleviation of human suffering as of

the highest importance, he feels that his first and greatest
work is to bring the Gospel to bear on the hearts and
consciences of the people. The patients assemble at an
early hour, and the work of the day is begun by holding
a service in the waiting-room. " Very pleasing it is,"
writes Dr. Christie, " to notice with what marked attention the patients listen to the Word preached, which tells
of the disease of sin, and of the Great Physician who is
able and willing to remove it. During the year, five have
been received into the Church by baptism, the first-fruits
of these services. Of these one is a literary man, with
a degree equivalent to our B.A., whose scholarship,
combined with earnestness, is calculated to make him a
great power for good among his fellow-countrymen.
Deeply grateful as we feel for direct results, perhaps
there is even greater cause for thankfulness, in the
progress that has been made in the way of disarming
prejudice, removing misapprehensions, and gaining the
confidence of the people. The indirect influence of
medical mission work in a land like this cannot be over-
estimated. It shows forth in a practical form Christianity's
highest and best principle, which is benevolence. Often
have we heard the remark, ' It must be a good doctrine
which does so much for suffering humanity.' "

The medical mission at Niigata, Japan, supported by
the Edinburgh Medical Missionary Society, till early in
1885, when it was taken over by the American Board
of Missions, has been in operation for the past ten

years. It affords a striking illustration of the value of medical missions as an auxiliary to evangelistic work. Previous to Dr. Palm's arrival there in 1875, Niigata was the only treaty port in Japan where no Protestant missionaries were at work. The success of his medical and surgical work soon won for him the confidence and gratitude of the people. He was heartily welcomed by the native physicians, and his instructions and assistance eagerly sought by them, while several, through his instrumentality, embraced Christianity, and became earnest, devoted fellow-labourers with him in the Gospel. When he left Niigata two years ago, he had the joy of seeing a native Christian church, with upwards of seventy communicants, which, under God, he had been the means of forming, and over which till his departure he presided; he had likewise established, in connection with the medical mission, fourteen preaching stations in the neighbouring towns and villages.

A good-sized volume might be filled with the interesting records of medical missionary work, its triumphs in India, China, Japan, Formosa, Siam, and Burmah; and not alone in these great mission fields, but also in Madagascar, Africa, Persia, Central Turkey, and Syria, in many parts of the continents of America and Europe, and in the cities throughout our own land where medical missions are in operation.

With one more illustration, we must pass on to review other aspects of the work. What we are about to relate takes us back to the beginning of the modern medical missionary enterprise. The narrative is associated with one whose name is well known, and who will ever be remembered as one of the pioneers of medical missions. We refer to Dr. Robert Kalley and his work in Madeira, which at the time was spoken of as "the greatest fact in modern missions."

Arrested in the midst of a gay and thoughtless career, through the effectual preaching of the Gospel, he was constrained by the love of Christ to devote his life to the Master's service as a missionary. Having finished his medical studies and graduated, Dr. Kalley at once offered himself to the London Missionary Society, and was accepted with the view of being sent to China. Meanwhile Mrs. Kalley's health gave way, and she was recommended to try a residence in a milder climate. Being in independent circumstances, Dr. Kalley resigned his connection with the missionary society, and in 1839 proceeded with Mrs. Kalley to Madeira. As soon as he was able to speak the Portuguese language, he opened a dispensary for the sick poor, and crowds came to him from all parts of the island for advice and medicine. To the assembled patients he read the Word of God, and preached the Gospel. Portions of the Bible in Portuguese were freely distributed, and many copies of the Holy Scriptures were readily purchased by his patients. Dr. Kalley invited inquirers to come to his own house for further instruction, and many availed themselves of the opportunity ; he was frequently asked to visit patients in the more distant towns and villages in the interior, where he had opportunities of proclaiming the Gospel in public places, and was eagerly listened to by large crowds. Like his Divine Master, he went about among the cities and villages, teaching and preaching and healing the sick, and like Him, he had soon to suffer for the testimony which he thus bore. By the blessing of God a deep impression was produced upon the minds of many who were previously bigoted Romanists, many began to question the infallibility of Rome, and not a few believed the simple truths of the Gospel, and were led to accept of Christ as their Saviour. This roused the indignation of the priesthood, who urged the public authorities to institute proceedings against Dr. Kalley, which ended in his being arrested and imprisoned, on a charge of "blasphemy and abetting heresy and apostacy." Early in 1844, through the interference of the British Government, he was set at liberty, and at once resumed his medical and evangelistic labours. He was soon made to feel, however, that a powerful enemy was at work against him. Several of his converts were seized and cast into prison, and he himself was again and again threatened with personal violence. Failing to obtain protection from the British authorities, he was at length obliged to escape for his life from the island. Notwithstanding all these untoward events, the good seed sown by Dr. Kalley, under the quickening influence of God's Holy Spirit, sprang up and yielded much fruit.   As the result of this movement, upwards of eight hundred persons threw off the yoke of Rome, who, being denied liberty in their own country to worship God according to the teaching of God's Word and the dictates of conscience, left their home and kindred, and founded for themselves a new colony, first in Trinidad, and ultimately in the Mississippi valley. After leaving Madeira, Dr. Kalley went to Malta, and there engaged in the same good work.   From thence he went to Syria, where his labours were much blessed, and after paying a visit to the Madeira refugees at Illinois, he settled in South America, where for many years he was greatly blessed in his work of healing the sick and preaching the Gospel.

Dr. Kalley is now resident in Edinburgh, and is one of the directors of the Edinburgh Medical Missionary Society, and we are indebted to him for the following deeply interesting incident, which he related at one of the meetings of the Society, and afterwards wrote out for us.   It is a striking illustration of the value or medical missionary work, as well as an encouragement to the Christian worker who is often cast down because of the little apparent fruit resulting from his labours.   It is also full of interest as a fulfilment of the Divine promise, " Cast thy bread upon the waters, for thou shalt find it after many days."   " In the morning sow thy seed, and in the evening withhold not thine hand ; for thou knowest not whether shall prosper either this or that, or whether they both shall be alike good.

"I spent 1850-52 in Syria," writes Dr. Kalley, "and during that time passed a summer on the Lebanon, in a village about 2000 feet above the sea level. While there I used to devote four or five hours daily to seeing the sick, and supplying them with medicine. Many came from far, and their eagerness in seeking relief helped me to form some idea of the crowds which gathered round Him who cured the leper with a touch, and raised the dead with a word.

"I seldom went to the houses of my patients, as the long mountain rides would have been too fatiguing for me, besides absorbing the time which was better employed in seeing and speaking with those who came to me. I, however, made an exception in the case of a young man employed in a silk factory belonging to a friend of mine. This youth's mother had ascites (dropsy), for which, along with other remedies, I repeatedly tapped her. Her son was present on these occasions, examined the trocar, and saw how the operation was performed. Shortly afterwards I went from Lebanon to Carmel, the plain of Esdraelon, &c. The poor woman continued to suffer much from the re-accumulation of the fluid, and her son (with true Arab self-confidence) ventured on having an instrument made, as like the trocar as he could, with which he operated upon his mother with his own hand, and succeeded.

"I left Syria soon after my return from the south, and did not see my patient again, neither did I hear any-

thing further about her son, till a few weeks ago, when I
received a letter from him, written in broken English by
one of his children. It is dated 1st December, 1883,
more than thirty-one years after our last interview. In
his letter he reminds me that I operated four times on
his mother, but says nothing of his own performance.
Then he adds, 'Your speaking to me was always from
the Gospel,' and 'I listened to your words, not because
I believed, but that you should attend my mother.' He
goes on to say that in 1852 (the year I left Syria) he
married. In 1854 he was appointed a Greek priest, and
continued to act as such 'with pleasure for eight years.'
During the ninth year, and till the seventeenth of his
priesthood, he says, 'Your sermons began to grow in my
heart.' After that his conscience obliged him to give
up his Greek priesthood. He commenced meetings for
Scriptural worship in his own house, and says he was
much persecuted, but the Lord was with him. He tells
me he has now been a Protestant teacher for ten years;
that for three years he has been working at Es-Salt, on
the east of the Jordan; then three years at Nazareth,
and in the villages around, and now resides in the village
where his mother lived. About forty meet for worship in
his house, and twelve are communicants. He writes,
'Your words which you put in my heart were buried so
many years, then they grew, and became, by God's grace,
a large tree, which flourishes, and will continue to flourish,
and bring forth fruit by the power of God.' He adds,

' You must know, that when I heard you were still alive, my joy was as Joseph's joy when he heard that his father was alive ; but oh ! from where shall I bring the carriages to send for you ? ' "

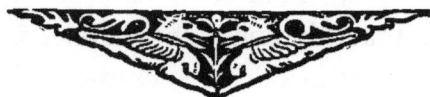

# THE NEED OF MEDICAL MISSIONS IN OUR MISSION FIELDS ABROAD.

## CHAPTER VI.

### The need of Medical Missions in our Mission Fields abroad. The claims of the Heathen, of our Converts, and of the Mission Families.

THE Christ-like nature of medical missionary work, the opportunities which it affords for the practical manifestation of the spirit of the Gospel—the doors, otherwise closed, which it opens in pioneering a way for the entrance of the truth—these are features of this department of work which cannot fail, if intelligently apprehended, to commend the cause to the hearty sympathy and support of the friends of missions.

Besides these, however, there are many important considerations which enhance the value of medical missions, and strengthen our plea for their more general employment in the foreign field. First of all, there is the lamentable ignorance existing in all heathen communities as to the cause, prevention, and cure of disease, which necessarily implies a fearful amount of preventible suffering and mortality. This ignorance is a fruitful source of superstition, and, consequently, one of the most effectual barriers in such lands to the uprooting of idolatrous rites and ceremonies.

In India, China, Africa, Madagascar, and in almost every heathen land, crude systems of medicine are intimately associated with the religions of the people, and the treatment of disease, such as it is, is monopolized by the priests, or by others under their control. The existence and prevalence of disease of every kind are ascribed to the agency of evil spirits, or to the anger of the gods; and unless these spirits and offended deities are propitiated, the direst results are foretold. The Hindoo Shastras, for instance, teach that any person rejecting the services of one of the native Hakims, or physicians, in time of sickness will, if the disease prove fatal, suffer inconceivable misery in the next world; whereas if a Hakim be employed, and the prescribed rites performed, the patient will be sure to go to heaven, even should he not be able to see the Ganges in his dying moments. As the result of such ignorance and superstition, one of the greatest trials which the missionary meets with in his work is the apostacy, in time of sickness, of not a few of his hopeful converts. Nor is this to be wondered at, when we remember that the only pretender to a knowledge of disease and its cure which the convert has ever known, is the unprincipled charlatan, the native physician, with his mantrams, charms, and propitiatory offerings. Deluded by the artful pretensions of the priest-physician, or urged by the entreaties of heathen relatives and friends, or overcome by his former superstitious fears, it too often happens, at such a time, that the weak professor allows heathen rites to be performed, and makes vows which, on recovery, he is compelled to perform, and thus, at the very outset, makes shipwreck of his faith.

In Madagascar, even in the immediate neighbourhood of the capital, and where the Gospel has won such triumphs, the power of former superstitions is still very manifest, especially among the older portion of the population. When sickness or trouble of any kind arises in their families, we find the Malagasy converts but too easily seduced into their old heathen ways. One missionary, after reporting the devastating effects of a severe epidemic among his people, writes: "This fearful disease threw back many of the natives upon their old superstitious rites and customs. It was a time of severe trial, and much of our work could not stand this crucial test. The people sought after 'wizards that peep and that mutter,' and ceased to seek unto their God. For a season, there was a strong current of idolatry and witchcraft running throughout the district, and many went back from their faith. Everywhere the churches were emptied of worshippers, and the schools of scholars, while the charm-maker found his enchantments eagerly sought after and liberally paid for. The most absurd things were done to effect cures by the orders of these diviners, and again and again during this sad time my own eyes beheld things which showed unmistakably what a powerful reaction had set in."

Another of the Imerina missionaries, writing on this subject, says : " The most serious effect of the epidemic was to drive multitudes of the people back to their old heathen practices, with the hope of charming away the disease. I was once led by a native pastor to the summit of a lofty hill, and there, amidst a grove of trees, was pointed out to me a rude kind of altar, where the blood of animals and fowls was spilt, and offerings of honey and bits of silver were constantly made, to assuage the anger of the spirits which were supposed to have brought the fever. I was told that it was an almost daily resort of the people, and that, on the Sabbath, some even of the Christians would gather round the table of the Lord, in remembrance of the blood 'shed for many for the remission of sins,' and on the afternoon of the same day would assemble in the 'sacred grove,' to present a sacrifice of blood to the spirits of their deceased ancestors."

We have referred to the sad influence of former superstitions among the Malagasy converts, who have so recently emerged from the darkness of heathenism ; but we must remember that, in this respect, they are not by any means singular ; indeed, in all our mission fields, wherever the great proportion of the people are still heathen, we may expect to find the same evil influences at work. We can testify from personal knowledge, that in Southern India this is one of the most common snares to the native Christian adherents, and, to some extent, even to the communicant, exerting a most powerful influence, and constantly calling for the exercise of church discipline; and hence, a very serious question arises: Are we dealing fairly with our converts from heathenism, when we subject them to church discipline for availing themselves in time of sickness of the only help within their reach, and on which, in their heathen state, they placed unbounded confidence, while we fail to provide them with necessary medical aid? It is not their blame that heathen rites and ceremonies are associated with the native treatment of disease, and they must either submit to the superstitious ordeal, or resist the entreaties of relatives and friends, and so suffer cruel neglect, or bring upon themselves their dire maledictions. If we remember these circumstances—the heathen influence all around, from the bondage of which they have so recently escaped, we shall, perhaps, in this matter be disposed to censure them with a little less severity.

We protest, and we cannot do so too strongly, against a system of Government education in India which, while it necessarily undermines the cherished religion of our fellow-subjects, not only does not provide, but actually prohibits the teaching of a better and a purer faith. In our aggressive missionary work, however, are we not doing a like injustice to this people? We deny to our converts the only help they can command, a help on which, from their earliest years, they have been taught implicitly to rely in time of affliction, and yet we provide no better aid for them. The importance of recognizing the healing art as the handmaid of religion is therefore very plainly indicated, in view of the claims of our native Christians gathered out of heathenism. What has thus been joined together, and forms part of almost every heathen system of religion, let us not put asunder; rather, from the usage of heathen nations, as well as from the practice and precept of Christ Himself and His disciples, let the Christian Church learn the lesson, that sanctified medical skill should go hand in hand with the Gospel in her evangelistic work.

In view of the plea we are urging, too much importance cannot be attached to the department of medical missionary work, which Dr. Valentine has done so much to promote in Northern India—which the late Dr. Paterson and Dr. Elder, in Madras, Dr. Green in Ceylon, and which we ourselves, and our successor, in Travancore, have each successfully prosecuted—namely, the training of intelligent native Christian youths to serve as medical evangelists to their fellow-countrymen. Just in proportion as such native medical agency is available throughout our mission districts, will the evil to which we have alluded, humanly speaking, be removed.

It will be seen from the foregoing, that all barbarous and semi-civilized nations are ignorant of the fundamental principles of medical science. Common humanity, therefore, to say nothing of Christian benevolence, should surely prompt to the adoption of means, whereby the mercenary and heartless pretensions of the priest-physicians may be exposed, the sick and suffering be cared for and comforted, and the cruelties inflicted upon them mitigated.

Some illustrations of the heathen principles and practice of medicine will show the need there is for medical mission agency.

The Chinese have a very extensive medical literature, but no works on anatomy or physiology. The kind of teaching imparted may be gathered from the following description of the pulse in its relation to disease : "There are three pulses in each wrist. A man's strongest pulse is in his left wrist, a woman's in her right. In a man, the pulse that lies nearest the hand is stronger than those that lie above ; in a woman just the opposite is true. In the left hand are located the pulses showing the diseases of the heart, the liver, and the kidneys, while the right hand pulses indicate the diseases of the lungs, the spleen, and other organs."

In one of their books, considered a great authority on the nature of disease, we read that the elements which compose the human body are fire, earth, iron, water, and wood. So long as the equilibrium of these is main-

tained, people enjoy health, but as soon as one pre-
dominates, sickness ensues.   All disease is therefore but
a disturbance of this equilibrium, and the art of healing
consists in restoring the balance.

The usual way for a Chinaman to enter the profession
is to procure a pair of spectacles with large bone rims,
some grasses and herbs, an assortment of spiders, and a
few venomous snakes, which he places in bottles in his
shop window.   Here is one of his prescriptions—

> " Powdered snakes    ...    2 parts.
>   Wasps and their nests   1 part.
>   Centipedes    ...    ...    6 parts.
>   Scorpions...    ...    ...    4    ,,
>   Toads    ...    20    ,,

Grind thoroughly, mix with honey, and make into small
pills.   Two to be taken four times a day."   In cases of
debility, the bones of the tiger, reduced to powder and
made into pills, are administered as a tonic.   They
reason thus: the tiger is very strong, the bone is the
strongest part of the strong animal—therefore, a pill of
this must be pre-eminently strengthening.

Dr. Hobson, for many years a medical missionary in
China, and author of several valuable works on medicine,
thus writes: "Medical science in China is at a low ebb.
It does not equal the state of the medical art in the time
of Hippocrates and Celsus.   The knowledge of anatomy
and surgery in ancient Greece and Rome was much

superior to anything now in China. At present there are no colleges or schools in the country, excepting the Imperial College at Pekin, for the use of his Majesty and high officers. Anatomy is totally interdicted, both by law and public opinion. Any man, however, may practise medicine, and thousands do so with the slender knowledge which their books afford. In these books, which are based on principles adopted two or three thousand years ago, the important doctrine of the circulation of the blood is not only not understood, but preposterously confused and erroneous. Their theory of the pulse proves this to a demonstration. There is no distinction between the arteries and veins, no knowledge of the heart's proper function, nor of the changes which the blood undergoes in the lungs and capillary system. The Chinese know nothing of the nervous system, its functions and diseases. They have a pulse for every organ but the brain. The position, forms, and uses of the viscera are not understood. There is no lack of books and observations on the functions of the body ; for everything, even the most inscrutable and mysterious, is explained by the *Yin* and the *Yang*—the hot and the cold, the dry and the moist, the superior and inferior influences ! Almost every symptom is a disease, and every prescription, of which the books contain thousands, is for every imaginable symptom, indicating a miserably small acquaintance with the nature and causes of disease."

Under such circumstances of ignorance and superstition, it is not wonderful that the mortality of China is very heavy. It is said that the daily mortality is not less than 33,000. When an epidemic breaks out, the people die by hundreds. The only remedy in times of plague or pestilence that they know, is to organize a series of Buddhistic services to expel the evil spirits supposed to be the cause of the calamity. We, in England, have had our age of superstition and ignorance, with reference to the causes of disease and the remedies. The light of Heaven has shone in on our darkness, and, under the influence of a free and pure Christianity, medical science has long been teaching us how to mitigate suffering and save life. The helpless condition of the Chinese in the face of disease or physical suffering is surely, in the light of the life of Jesus Christ, a call to us to give them a share of the blessing that God has given to us.

Dr. Sturge, medical missionary in Siam, gives an interesting account of the Siamese theory and practice of medicine. All nature, according to the Siamese, is made up of four elements, namely, fire, earth, wind, and water. The human body is supposed to be composed of the same elements, which they divide into two classes, visible and invisible. To the former, belongs everything that can be seen, as the bones, flesh, blood, &c; to the latter, the wind and the fire. The body is composed of twenty kinds of earth, twelve kinds of water, six kinds of wind, and four kinds of fire. The varieties of wind are as follows : the first kind passes from the head to the feet, and the second variety from the feet to the head ; the third variety resides about the diaphragm, and the fourth circulates in the arteries forming the pulse ; the fifth enters the lungs, and the sixth resides in the intestines. The four kinds of fire are, first, that which gives the body its natural temperature ; the second, that which causes a higher temperature, as after exercise or in fevers ; the third variety causes digestion, and the fourth causes old age. The Siamese divide the body into thirty-two parts, as the skin, heart, lungs, &c. The body is subject to ninety-six diseases, due to the disarrangement of the earth, wind, fire, and water. Thus, if there is an undue proportion of fire, we have one of the fevers. Dropsies are caused by too great a proportion of water, and wind causes all manner of complaints. Nine out of ten of the natives, when asked what is the matter with them, answer " Wind."

Spirits are supposed to have great power over our bodies, deranging the elements and producing all manner of diseases. The minds of the natives are thus held in continual bondage for fear of the spirits, for no one knows what great sins he may have committed in a previous state of existence, for which he may be called upon to suffer at any moment. Thus the people are constantly endeavouring to propitiate them by presents, incantations, &c.

With regard to medicines, they believe that in the time of Buddha, there lived one still worshipped as the Father of Medicine. To him, it is said, the plants all spoke, telling their names and medicinal properties. These were written in books, and have become sacred. If they fail to produce the effects attributed to them, the fault is not theirs, but the want of success is due to the absence of merit in either doctor or patient. The natives use almost everything as medicine ; the bones and skins of various animals occupy a large part of their pharmacopœia, while the galls of snakes, tigers, lizards, &c., are among the most valuable of their remedies. The following is a most absurd recipe for the bite of a snake : 'A portion of the jaw of a wild hog, a portion of the jaw of a tame hog, a portion of the jaw of a goat, a portion of goose bone, a portion of peacock bone, a portion of the tail of a fish, and a portion of the head of a venomous snake.' These being duly compounded, form a popular remedy when the venom has caused lockjaw. Many other remedies are equally foolish. Every native physician has an image of the Father of Medicine in his house. The drugs are placed in the idol's hand, and receive his blessing ; afterwards they are taken to the patient's house and boiled in earthen pots, a wicker-work star being placed below and above the drugs to give the medicine strength.

In India, notwithstanding the progress of Western science, the condition of the people, with regard to disease and its treatment, is barbarous beyond description.

"Bound hand and foot by the fetters of superstition," writes the Rev. W. Shoolbred, "a rude stone, bedaubed with red paint, oil, or ghee, without even the semblance of anything in heaven, earth, or the waters under the earth, represents their deity; and the virtues supposed to reside in that stone are inexhaustible. Is a man sick, he has only to go to the nearest temple, or to the rude stone beneath the village tree, worship and present the usual offerings. Enough; let him wait and he will be healed. Some of the representatives of Kheturpal (one of the gods worshipped by the hill people in the Mairwara district) are much more potent in healing diseases or averting evil than the others. Thus the one in a small temple at Shamgurh is supposed to be espècially efficacious. I found a poor farmer, lame and crippled from rheumatism, lying before this temple door. He had been there for more than two months, waiting for a cure, but as yet in vain."

"The common people in Western India," writes the Rev. R. A. Hume, Ahmednagar, "think that cholera is a punishment sent on men by an evil goddess. As they suppose that it would offend her to call her a bad name, she is called *Murree Ai*, that is, Cholera Mother. They also think that giving and taking medicine for the disease only excites the Mother still more, and that the only proper way to get rid of the pestilence is to honour the Mother, and so induce her to go elsewhere. In all the villages, there are one or two small temples dedicated to the Cholera Mother, in which there are a few shapeless stones painted red. These temples are built near the extreme limits of the town, so that the goddess may stay far from the houses of the people. At the time of an epidemic these are repaired. In most towns there are a few men and women of the lowest castes who are devotees of this goddess, and when cholera is prevalent they get much attention and much profit. Even intelligent men come and ask these ignorant devotees, 'What is the Mother's pleasure ? How long does she intend to favour the town with her presence, and what can we do for her?' Then the devotee pretends to go into a kind of trance, and, after a shaking fit, replies that the Mother says that she intends to remain for so many days, and would like such and such attentions. These attentions the people gladly show."

Among the millions of devil-worshippers in Southern India, the following legendary tale accounts for the existence of disease, and indicates the source of deliverance. On a certain day, when celestial food was carried to Siva by some of the inferior gods, the giant Taradan overpowered them, and seizing the repast, devoured it. Siva became very angry at the loss of his meal, and determined to punish the offender. He created the sacred Vedas for the assistance of Pattera-Kalee and Veerapatteram, and delivered them into their hands along with a trident, Siva's emblem and instrument of destruction, directing them to make war with Taradan.

They executed their commissions so promptly and effectually, that Siva's enemy was destroyed, to his great delight. Siva was so pleased with their success that he endowed them with unlimited power to inflict all manner of disease, and to kill all on earth who opposed them, or neglected to offer sacrifices at their altars. The consequence was, that many were killed, or grievously afflicted with terrible diseases. This produced great consternation, and led the people to inquire of the priests as to the origin, and the means to be adopted for the removal of these calamities, and they informed them, that although Siva had given the demons the dreadful power which they were exercising, still they might be propitiated if they would offer sacrifices at their shrines; festivals were accordingly established, at which bloody sacrifices of sheep, goats, and fowls, with plantains, flowers, and incense, were to be offered, and those who joined in these, and similar ceremonies, were promised protection or deliverance if afflicted with disease. We have been present on several occasions, and the scenes we witnessed were sickening and humiliating beyond description. At the Mundycadu festival, thousands from all parts of Travancore and Tinnevelly assembled to fulfil the vows they had made in time of sickness. Outside of the pagoda a large quantity of cocoanuts and other offerings is piled up; also a heterogeneous heap of wooden hands, arms, legs, and feet, offered by those who have been restored from some injury or disease in those members; rich convalescents present silver models of hands and legs, or even golden ones on such occasions—these, however, are carefully put away within the temple. In one direction, persons may be seen rolling naked in the dust for several hours at a time, until, exhausted by the heat and exertion, they faint and are carried off, more like huge unshapely masses of mud than human beings; others, have a long supple piece of cane inserted through folds of flesh in their sides, crossed over their chest, and pass along maddened with the pain and excitement, while one behind keeps step, jerking the cane backwards and forwards through the raw bleeding wounds. Parents and relations may be seen bringing forward scores of children of both sexes, to have this cruel rite performed upon them, in fulfilment of vows made on their behalf while suffering from some sickness; here and there others may be seen with little earthenware vessels full of burning charcoal placed on their naked chests, and allowing it to remain there till the flesh on the breast is actually roasting beneath, hoping in this way to propitiate the anger of the evil spirits they so much dread, and gain immunity from the disease that threatens to afflict them.

In the *Antananarivo Annual*, No. VI., an interesting account is given, by the Rev. A. Walen, of the superstitions, religious ideas, and ceremonies of the Sakalava, on the west coast of Madagascar. They believe in the existence of a superior Being, whom they called Andrianânahàry, which means the " creating and arranging prince," who is the object of the Sakalava's fear, but not of their love and desire. They believe in a duality of character, or the existence of good and evil, in God. These different qualities are not concentrated in different persons or beings who are in a state of opposition or conflict, but are blended in one individual, and their possessor makes use of them according to his inclination. "They regard God as the ruler over life and death; but there are also other beings beside God who cause death. The ancestors and *ampamàrike* (wizards) have power to bring about the death of any one. If, therefore, a person becomes ill, his relations first of all go to ask the *ampisikily* (diviners) whether the sickness will end in death or not. The first answer is always equivocal, for the Sakalava know well how to make a statement that may bear two meanings. Being asked for further information as to who causes the sickness, the diviner replies, perhaps it is caused by God, and that He is now about to cause the death of the individual in question, and so his relations prepare means to avert the dreadful calamity. They immediately send for an ox; if they have none themselves they are obliged to buy one, which must be small and in poor condition, and the cheaper the better. When the ox is procured, the relations and friends of the sick man gather together and form a circle, in the middle of which the victim is placed. A small altar is built which is called *vavàra;* the head of the family then advances towards the victim, and repeats a form of prayer

in which he, before God, complains of their present misfortune, death having approached the family.   On this
account they are in deep distress and terror, says he, and
therefore yield the life of an ox, which they offer to Him
as a gift instead of the human life.   Thereupon the
victim is killed; the head of the family gives the first stab,
and the others go on sticking, spearing, cutting, and
carving the poor animal in a dreadful manner until it is
dead.   It is then cut up without being flayed, for to skin
a victim would be considered a cardinal sin against the
law of the ancestors.   The people now prepare their pots
for cooking, while the sacrificer takes the suet, and puts
it either on a kind of gridiron or on the fire, burning it
on the *vavàra* (altar) in order that it shall ascend to
Andrianànahàry as an acceptable incense.   After this
the flesh is cooked and eaten ; small pieces of the meat
are sent as presents to those of the friends of the family
who were not present at the sacrificial banquet, and the
feast comes to an end.   In lieu of cattle, rum may be
used as an offering.   In this case the persons divide the
rum into two portions, one for themselves, and one for
Andrianànahàry.   Their own portion they of course
swallow at once, that belonging to God being poured out
on the ground."

Mr. R. W. Felkin, F.R.S.E., F.R.G.S., in "Notes on the
Madi or Moru tribe of Central Africa," published in the
Proceedings of the Royal Society, Edinburgh, Vol. XII.,
1883–84, gives details regarding the social condition,

manners, and customs of this tribe, of much value and interest to those engaged in the study of anthropology. As to the practice of medicine and surgery among the Madis, Mr. Felkin tells us that there are male and female doctors, the males confining their practice to wounds, accidents, and snake bites. The treatment of a broken arm or leg is noteworthy. When it is a simple fracture, the limb is pulled as straight as possible, and then sticks are placed as splints to keep it in position, and are tied with cords. When the bone is broken in pieces, and the limb swells so that they cannot properly straighten it, a number of small cuts are made, and cupping horns applied; when the swelling has been reduced, if still unable to straighten the limb, they cut the broken bones out, and fix on splints, applying a powdered root to the wound. Hæmorrhage is stopped by actual cautery (a red-hot iron). This operation is rarely successful—most people who undergo it die in a few days. Women doctors treat all cases except those mentioned above. They have but few medicines, and seem to make frequent use of magic. When a woman doctor is called to visit a patient, she brings with her a basket containing what she calls her magic wand—a kind of double tube about a foot long, each tube being about four inches in diameter. The one tube is partly filled with small stones, the other is empty, to allow of the doctor performing her manipulations in it. This instrument is painted red, and oiled all over. The doctor shakes the wand, and mutters to

herself for some little time; then feels the patient all over,
and draws her wand over him.   When pain is complained
of in the abdomen or chest, she first rubs the part with
oil, and then places her wand over the painful spot,
introducing her hand into the empty tube.   After working about for some time, she at last draws out a
substance which she calls the disease, taking care that
the people shall not have any opportunity of seeing it
closely.   If pain is felt in the head, she cups the patient
on the temples or nape of the neck, by making small
cuts with a stone; an iron knife is not used. . . . There
appears to be a belief in the existence of elves, or spirits,
though this would seem to be an invention of the female
doctors to gain a hold on the people.   "Odi" is the
name by which these beings are known.   They are
supposed to live underground, and their help is sought in
cases of illness among children.   If a child is ill, the lady
doctor first examines it, and then retires to a quiet spot
at a distance from the hut, where she erects a miniature
hut of sticks and grass.   She is followed to this place by
the mother and one of her little boys, laden with a pot
of food and a live fowl.   She then proceeds to invoke
the Odi to appear, but often gives out that they cannot
come till next day, being busy.   At last they make their
appearance inside the hut, but are visible to none but the
doctor, others only hearing them speak.   Two usually
appear, a male and a female, more than that number
refusing to come at once.   The doctor says they have

human faces and serpents' bodies. She pretends to give them food to eat out of the pot, and asks their aid toward the sick child's recovery, shaking all the time her magic wand or rattle. When they have enough food they vanish, and the doctor falls down right over the small hut. She strikes the ground with her hand, and appears to have a fit, unconsciousness lasting a few minutes. Before falling, she tells the mother and boy to run home as fast as possible, and shut the door. A strong woman is always present at this incantation, who is ready to raise the fallen doctor, and gives her water to drink. After she has recovered from her real or supposed exhaustion, she is supported to the sick child's hut to see her patient. Before the door is opened a certain formula is gone through, after which she enters the hut, feels the child all over, and gives her opinion as to whether it will get well or not. She is then escorted home by the father, who takes with him her fee, in the shape of a goat, cow, or arrows.

Mr. J. T. Last, of the Church Missionary Society's Eastern Central African Mission, relates the following incident, which painfully illustrates the terrible superstition of the people, and the extreme cruelty into which their fancies lead them. "About twelve months ago, Msamwenda, the chief of the village of Kirabi, had a son born to him. Not quite a month ago, Msamwenda came to me with a sorrowful face, and after the usual salutations, I asked him what was amiss. He told me that his child had cut its upper teeth first, and that the people were demanding that it should be thrown into the forest, where it would be eaten by the hyenas.   They make this demand on the ground that, if a *Mgego* (a child who cuts its upper teeth first) is allowed to live, it will cause the death of all the great men of the place.   Msamwenda refused to comply with this request, until he heard what I had to say in the matter.   He was in tears when he told me about his child, but when I told him we had no sympathy with such cruelty, and that he must not destroy God's gift in such a manner, he dried his tears, and said he would not throw away his child, even though it should cost him his life.   After he had some more talk with the natives, the matter dropped.   But now the death of two chiefs since Msamwenda came to me has raised again the cry against the child.   A short time ago the chief of Bwagamoyo, Rufus by name, was killed by the Wahwmba, and now Malundo has been accidentally shot, and the superstitious natives believe that it must be through the influence of the *Mgego.*   Yesterday morning Msamwenda came to me, and begged me to take the child to Zanzibar, and have it brought up as a Christian.   'The people here,' he said, 'were all craving for it to be killed, and he could not kill his own child, nor allow others to do so.' After considering the case, and in the hope that the child, being so brought up apart from all native super-stitions may become a good and useful man, I con-sented to take him to Zanzibar, and do my best for him."

Not infrequently, the natives of the Friendly Islands, in order to check any spreading ulceration or disease, hack off the limb at a joint, working a sharp shell to and fro and making a horribly jagged wound. In cases of delirium the patient is invariably buried alive, and it is related how a young man, in the prime of life, was twice buried, and in his frenzy twice burst up the grave ; he was afterwards lashed to a tree and allowed to die of starvation.

Among the natives of the South Pacific Islands, " cutting " is the universal remedy for every ailment. If pain in the head is felt, then an incision, or perhaps two, is made over the part " to let the pain out ;" if diarrhœa is the complaint, then cuts are made over the abdomen ; if rheumatism, deep incisions are made over the part affected ; if fever, various parts of the body are cut.

It would be easy to multiply instances of the ignorant, barbarous, and superstitious notions of the people in all heathen lands, with respect to the nature and cause, the treatment and prevention, of disease, but the foregoing will give some conception of the need there is for the beneficent ministry of the missionary physician. No friend of humanity, and surely no friend of missions, can think of such heathenish rites and ceremonies performed over the sick and dying, of the cruel ordeals imposed upon them and the untold sufferings inflicted, and of the holocausts of victims thereby consigned to an untimely death, without endeavouring to stretch forth a helping hand to ameliorate their sad condition. What an honour would be conferred upon the Church were she to avail herself of the privilege, and be the instrument of carrying the blessings of our great modern discoveries, and the improvements in medical and surgical science, along with the Gospel, into those distant and barbarous lands, where humanity languishes and suffers under the agonies of unmitigated disease !

But besides the claims of the heathen, and of those from amongst them who are led to embrace Christianity, and by so doing profess to renounce all reliance and participation in heathen rites and ceremonies, there are the claims of the missionaries themselves and of their families. We ask how far the Directors of our missionary societies are justified in sending forth young missionaries, either single or married, to settle down in untried and often unhealthy regions, without providing for them competent medical aid ? Parents, in giving up their sons and their daughters to go forth in the service of the Church as missionaries, would not be asking more than they have a right to expect, were they to insist upon such provision being made ; nor would the missionaries themselves be manifesting less faith, courage, and devotion. For our military expeditions, and commercial enterprises in foreign lands, alike from an economical point of view, and in justice to those engaged in them, medical aid and appliances are deemed indispensable, and are ungrudgingly supplied, and why should it be otherwise in the

missionary enterprise? No doubt our missionaries are
the very special objects of God's protection and care, as
the records of their lives testify; but we are not therefore relieved of our responsibility, when we rest contented
with merely commending them to the Divine protection,
and leave them destitute of that skilled medical aid
which, sooner or later, they will so much need.

We admire the faith, the courage, and the devotion of
those who, as the " Messengers of the Churches," have
gone forth, often to unhealthy and inhospitable climes,
renouncing the comforts and refinements of home and
of civilized society; and, not knowing the things that shall
befall them, have said with the Apostle, " But none of
these things move me, neither count I my life dear unto
myself, so that I might finish my course with joy, and the
ministry which I have received of the Lord Jesus, to
testify of the grace of God." Let us thank God, that
among the young men and women in our churches, there
exists so much of this spirit of self-sacrificing devotion;
may it increase and abound! But the very existence of
this noble, heroic missionary spirit, lays the Church
under deep obligation to provide for the conservation of
the health and the lives of her missionaries and their
families. Among the many blessings and privileges
which, for Christ's sake, they have surrendered, when the
" dark and cloudy day " of affliction comes, perhaps the
loss most keenly felt is the want of that kind, unre-
mitting medical skill and help which, more needed

abroad, is there all unknown. We often read in missionary reports of the illness and death of some devoted
missionary, or missionary's wife or child, in the interior of
Africa, it may be, or on the malarious plains of India or
China, or in some of the lonely islands of the sea.
There, in that solitary home, far, far away from kindred
and friends, in a strange land, with no skilled hand near
to administer relief, the life of the loved one ebbs away.
Let us picture to ourselves, if we can, the affecting realities
of such a scene of domestic missionary life—the feeling of
utter helplessness and desolation, the crushed hopes, the
blasted prospects, the breaking hearts, the heavy sorrow,
in such an hour, of the inmates of that lonely mission
dwelling, aggravated perhaps by the thought that,
had the skilled hand been near, with God's blessing
resting upon it, life and health and hope would have
come smiling back ! Such scenes, alas ! too often recorded, give painful emphasis to the appeal of a missionary who, in losing the wife of his youth under most
painful and trying circumstances, which, had medical aid
been within reach (as we hold it ought to be wherever
the Church sends her missionaries with their wives and
families), this valuable life in all human probability would
have been saved, was heard to say that he, with his
motherless babe in his arms, "would fain stand by her
lonely grave and lift up an earnest appeal for medical
missionaries to co-operate with them in their labours of
love, and to tend them and their loved ones in times of

sickness, till it was heard all over his native land, and responded to by the Church of Christ."

The idea is, we fear, too prevalent that missions to the heathen are altogether exempt from the conditions which determine the success or failure of ordinary human undertakings, and that in the prosecution of the missionary enterprise, we may therefore, to a large extent, depend upon a special providence to shield our missionaries, and dispense with much that in other circumstances would be deemed essential to success. Doubtless, missionary work is pre-eminently Divine, and its success the fruit of the Divine blessing ; but we have no right to presume that therefore, independently of all human precautions and the use of all available means, God will work miracles for the preservation of the health and lives of our brethren. "Have faith in God," is the Church's grand motto in view of her missionary obligations, but alike for personal salvation, and for security in the midst of danger, our faith must be a living principle ; and if our faith prompts to no earnest endeavour to provide "those things which are needful to the body," "what doth it profit? "

The medical care of the missionaries and their families forms no small nor unimportant part of the duty of the missionary physician, and the advantage of having a medical department in connection with a localized mission, from an economical point of view, as well as in the interests of the work and the comfort and the welfare of the missionaries, can hardly be over-estimated. We know of missionaries who, when reduced to extreme weakness by sickness, have been compelled to leave their stations, and take a journey of two or three hundred miles, in order to obtain the nearest medical aid, thereby not only incurring great risks, but also heavy expenses, and probably protracted absence from their work. Missionaries, too, owing to the temporary failure of their own, or their wives' health, have relinquished foreign service, who, had timely medical assistance been available, would probably have been still actively engaged in their loved work.

In view, then, of our obligations to the heathen and to those gathered out of heathenism ; for the sake of the missionaries themselves and their families, as well as from an economical point of view, we plead for the more general employment of this agency, and with so many thoroughly qualified and devoted young medical missionaries either offering themselves, or in course of preparation for this department of service, we hold that it is incumbent upon the Directors of our missionary societies to appoint missionary physicians wherever they plant their missions, and especially so in all the more isolated fields of labour. We believe, moreover, that the hearty sympathy of the constituents of our societies would support them in so doing.

# ZENANA MEDICAL MISSIONS.

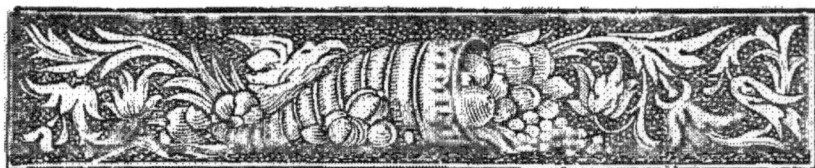

## CHAPTER VII.

### The qualifications, training, and position of the Female Medical Missionary.

"OH, if we could only get within these prisons of Zenanas!" wrote the late Dr. Elmslie of Kashmir, "if we could only emancipate their benighted tenants, and lead them forth into the glorious liberty of the Gospel!—then might we look with confidence for the speedy dawning of a bright day on India's countless sons;" and the Rev. Dr. Duff, in a letter we received from him shortly before his death, along with a copy of Dr. Elmslie's "Plea for Zenana Medical Missions," pleads most earnestly for something to be done in the direction indicated by Dr. Elmslie. "Every educated person," writes Dr. Duff, "knows the peculiar position of Hindu females of the upper classes, and how entirely they are secluded, and how, in their case, a male missionary might find no access to them. But if a female missionary knew something of medical science and practice, readily would *she* find access, and while applying her medical skill to the healing of the body, would have precious opportunities of applying the balm of spiritual healing to the worse diseases of the soul. Would to God we had such an agency ready for work ! Soon might India be moved in its innermost recesses !"

So much has been written within these last few years regarding the condition of woman in heathen lands, that it is scarcely necessary here to describe at any length their pitiable circumstances. It is well known that, so far as a knowledge of the laws of health, or of proper treatment in time of sickness is concerned, they are, as a rule, without either care or cure. Dr. C. R. Francis, whose professional experience in India extended over thirty years, writes: "An incredible number of, humanly speaking, preventible deaths occur every year among the many millions of Her Majesty's female subjects in this so-called gem of the Indian Empire. Native midwifery, in the ordinary meaning of the term, does not exist in India. Native surgery is of the most primitive kind. Hygiene, or preventive medicine, is utterly unknown. Some idea of the gross ignorance that prevails may be formed, when one hears that the women's apartments, in which many pairs of lungs are at work, represent at night a miniature "black-hole" of Calcutta ; that the accumulated house filth of every description is deposited in the immediate neighbourhood of the dwelling; and that, after child-birth, every breath of pure air is excluded from the lying-in chamber, which is kept almost hermetically sealed till the twenty-first day, when a religious ceremony known as *shoostee pooja* is performed." "All Hindu women," writes Mrs. Weitbrecht, the well-known Zenana missionary, "whether rich or poor, are utterly neglected in the time of sickness. Prejudices and customs banish medical aid altogether; infectious and other diseases are left to take their own course. Two thousand children, not very long ago, were left to perish from small-pox in one city. A female medical mission in every populous centre is one of the most crying needs of India; an agency which would find its way into those dark, dirty, miserable dwellings, where fever, ophthalmia, and other ills spread unchecked. The death-rate among women and children is enormous, and constant sickness is one of the greatest hindrances to the Zenana missionary."

"The real doctors of India," writes the late Dr. Elmslie, "are the native hakims, who abound everywhere, and are totally ignorant of Western medicine and surgery. Generally, the medical lore of both Hindu and Mussulman hakims consists of a few useless and disgusting nostrums, which have been handed down from sire to son for many generations. As to the diseases peculiar to women and children, they simply know nothing of them. Besides being ignorant, they are excessively meddlesome, and so do incalculable mischief when they are called in. How much England owes to her Simpsons, Priestleys, Farres, and Wests! India is now without such men, and, in her present state, could not and would not avail herself of them ; but she is ready, from the Himalayas to Cape Comorin, to receive with open arms any daughter of the West, who comes to assuage her pains and to bind up her wounds. Moreover, the native doctors are not generally called upon to treat the women of the Zenanas ; *when* they are called in, it is only to see the patient die, the time for doing anything hopefully efficacious having passed. Besides the native doctors or hakims, there is a numerous class of native nurses, who are, virtually, all the sick women of India have for doctors in their own homes. The native female nurses are generally very ignorant, meddlesome, and immoral. Very sad effects spring often from their gross ignorance and unlimited interference ; countless mothers and children fall victims. The death-rate amongst Indian women and children is enormous, and quite out of due proportion. Surely if these things are so, it is the duty of Christians in England, and especially of Christian women, to hold out a helping and sympathizing hand to their suffering Indian sisters."

While a medical missionary in India, we witnessed among the women, cases of heart-rending cruelty and neglect which we dare not describe ; cases in which, had medical aid been within reach at the proper time, humanly speaking, all would have gone well. Husbands have come to us imploring medicine for their wives who were dying of dysentery or fever—suffering untold agonies, the result, it might be, of some accident, or of the barbarous treatment of a native nurse; a not uncommon request was for some medicine to kill maggots in an open sore, and more than once we have been asked for ointment to heal the broken limb of some inmate of the Zenana; and when we told them in such cases that we must see the patient, and that perhaps some operation might be required, or that the broken bones must be set and the limb put in splints, "That cannot be, it is not our custom," has been the reply; and the poor woman has been left to linger on in suffering and misery, or die in her agony, simply for want of that help which the lady physician, or in many cases even the trained nurse, could have given.

What has been said of India is true of almost every Oriental country, and indeed of all lands on which the Gospel has not shed its Christianizing and humanizing influence. In these "dark places of the earth" woman is debased and neglected, and in the hour of her suffering and weakness, no skilled loving hand is stretched forth to administer the needed relief; and, as a rule, she will receive no help but from those of her own sex.

Much interest has recently been awakened on behalf of the women and children in our mission fields, especially those of India and China, and societies have been formed, in connection with almost every denomination, to promote this special department of service; and though the work of foreign female evangelization is as yet only in its infancy, still, by the blessing of God upon the efforts of the agents of these societies, wide and effectual doors have been opened, and an entrance gained into the secluded homes of the East. A most hopeful work has been inaugurated—a work which, ere long, will develop into much larger proportions, and occupy a much more prominent place amongst our mission agencies than it has yet done. As one branch of this work, Female Medical Missions cannot fail to secure the sympathy and support of all who have at heart the promotion of Zenana missions; indeed, so many requests are coming in—and from so many fields—for lady medical missionaries, and so many young ladies are now making inquiry as to the course of study, and the qualifications necessary for such service, that there is an evident interest awakened in this important subject.

A few words regarding the nature of female medical missionary work, the preliminary qualifications, as well as the subsequent training necessary for it, may therefore be helpful to those desiring to consecrate their lives to this Christ-like service.

We have, in a previous chapter, defined the sphere and function of the medical missionary, and that definition is equally applicable, whether the work is to be carried on by a lady physician, or by a medical man. Medical missions are established with the object not only of curing, but of Christianizing. The work of the female medical missionary is to heal the wounded and diseased body, that so, by her disinterested and benevolent services, she may overcome prejudice, soften bigotry, and dispel gloom; and while ministering relief to the suffering body, may thereby gain an entrance for the Gospel into the hearts and homes of her patients.

The first and most indispensable qualification in the candidate for this work is personal piety, and a hearty devotion and unreserved consecration to the service of her Lord and Master. There must be, as the constraining influence, a higher motive than the mere desire to engage in some useful service; the impelling motive must be "the love of Christ;" her heart must beat in true and ardent sympathy with Christ in His yearning solicitude for the salvation of the lost. In view of the trials, self-sacrifice, difficulties, and responsibilities of the work, she must feel as did the prophet when he said: "His word is in mine heart as a burning fire shut up in my bones, and I am weary with forbearing, and I cannot stay!" Unless her heart is fired with a genuine, steady, glowing love to her Saviour, with an earnest, enthusiastic desire for His glory, and an ardent longing for the salvation of souls, and, moreover, a proved capacity to influence and to convey truth to the minds of others, she had better not think of medical missionary service, nor, indeed, of any department of Christian work in the foreign field. Along with this indispensable qualification, there must be good mental abilities; a tender yet firm hand, and a kind, loving, sympathizing heart; common sense, or as the late Professor Miller expresses it, " *gump-tion;* " a bright, cheerful disposition ; ability and readiness to adapt herself to circumstances; great perseverance; a good, sound constitution ; strength of body and of mind to bear up under fatigue and anxiety, and, in some degree, a natural aptitude in acquiring a foreign language. It is difficult to fix the age at which preparation for Zenana medical missionary work should begin.    It is probable that, before commencing her purely medical studies, the candidate will require to devote a year or more to preparation for the preliminary examination in general education, which must be passed prior to registration as a medical student : but a lady, with foreign medical missionary work in view, should not, we think, begin her medical curriculum earlier than her twenty-first year, nor later than her twenty-fifth or twenty-sixth.

In the case of those whose circumstances prevent their taking a full course of medical study, and obtaining a license qualifying to practise—those, we mean, who must be content to serve as missionary nurses—while the same general qualifications are essential to success, the same high standard of education and of mental ability is not so necessary; nor will it be any drawback, if the age of such a candidate should be a little more advanced.

Amongst the friends of female medical mission work,

there is, we know, a difference of opinion as to the
extent of professional study, and the kind of medical
qualification necessary for this service; some believe
that a course of eighteen months' or two years' instruction and practical experience is quite sufficient, while
others hold that no one should undertake such a re‐
sponsible position, unless she has pursued a regular
course of medical study, and proved her efficiency by
obtaining a diploma or license to practise. In a certain
sense, both are right; in the great mission field, there is
room for the skilled Christian nurse, and a loud call for
her services, but there is as loud a call, and a still more
inviting and influential sphere of usefulness, for the
accomplished lady physician, and the one should be
as the complement of the other—indeed they ought to
work hand in hand. We have no hesitation in expressing most emphatically our conviction, that it is most
unadvisable to send out partially trained ladies to
undertake medical mission work on their own responsibility, and we believe that sooner or later the friends
of the cause will acknowledge this.

If a partially trained lady is sent out to practise
medicine among the women and children in the mission
field, if she calls herself a medical missionary, opens a
dispensary, and invites patients to come to her for healing, or offers to attend them at their own homes, of this
we are certain, she will not be long at work before she
will be called upon to treat cases, which will place her

in most painful and trying circumstances; and if, in
emergencies and cases of difficulty, she is unable to
render proper aid, her presence there will do the mission
cause more harm than good, and very likely her own
health will speedily break down under the terrible strain
of anxiety which, under such trying circumstances, she
must undergo. The partially trained agent, calling
herself a medical missionary, may depend upon it, that
the more successful she is in the treatment of ordinary
complaints, the more frequently she will be implored to
attend cases in presence of which she will stand powerless; and, unnerved by sufferings which she cannot
alleviate, and agitated by the sneers and, it may be, the
threats of ignorant by-standers, she will have good cause
to regret, that she ventured to accept a position for
which her training and qualifications never fitted her.

It is quite true that the aid such an one can give is
better than none, but that is not to the point; our con-
tention is, that it is wrong to send forth as medical
missionaries such agents to the mission field, and thereby
lead the natives to expect from them a greater, and more
skilled service, than they are able to render. From
medical missionaries, the heathen to whom they are sent
have a right to expect skilful aid, and especially will
they look for this in times of emergency, and when,
perhaps, all other help has failed. As a rule, the
accomplished lady physician will be able to render
the needed aid, and thereby, with God's blessing, gain

the confidence of the people, and open an avenue to the heart for the Gospel message ; but these are the very cases which the partially trained lady cannot treat, and hence, instead of winning the gratitude of the people, her inability to render help when most needed, may cause her good to be evil spoken of, and thus, her presence in the mission field, may really be more of a hindrance than a help.

We could adduce several instances confirmatory of what we have said ; one must suffice. A lady whom we knew well, the wife of a missionary in India, had, during her two years' furlough at home, availed herself of every opportunity to acquire a knowledge of medicine, and had enjoyed the personal friendship, and for six months the tuition, of the late Sir James Simpson. On returning to India, she made known throughout the district, that she was prepared to see patients at her own bungalow, and to visit women at their own homes, when they needed help. Not many days passed, till she was called to attend an expectant mother. The case was a very serious one, but just such a case as, over and over again, she had seen brought to a favourable termination, under skilful interference in the Maternity Hospital. Though quite competent to manage all ordinary cases, and even common emergencies, in presence of the complication she had now to deal with, she felt herself powerless. Unnerved by witnessing the suffering of the poor woman, without being able to render her any assistance, she left

the house, but not before the *dhais* (heathen nurse) had
prompted the priest to make it known to all, that the
mission doctor *amalé*, or lady, having been called in, the
gods were angry, and would not now be appeased.   Within
an hour the poor woman died; and after this sad experience, the lady suffered for months from such severe nervous
prostration, that more than once, before she could again
return to England, her life was despaired of.   This was
the first case, but also the last, in her *medical* missionary
experience, and, as can readily be believed, her effort in
that direction had no favourable influence on the work
of the mission.

Let us not be misunderstood.   There cannot be too
many thoroughly well-trained nurses sent out to work
amongst the women and children in our mission fields :
there is an urgent need for them, and, like our Bible-
women nurses at home, they will have splendid opportunities for sowing the good seed; but do not place
them in a position, or impose upon them duties, for
which they will quickly discover, that their professional
education and training never fitted them.   For their own
sakes, as well as for the sake of the cause we seek to
promote, do not designate as *medical missionaries* such
partially trained agents, and thus lead the inmates of the
Zenanas to expect from them services which they are not
qualified to render.   Do not instruct such agents to take
upon themselves the duties and responsibilities of a
doctor—to open a dispensary and a hospital—to invite

the sick and suffering to come to them for healing ; if they do, they must be prepared to receive all cases, urgent and simple, just as they come, and if they refuse cases of difficulty, and prove themselves, in the treatment of such cases, to be as powerless as the native *dhais* or hakim, what influence in favour of the mission can such an agency exert ?

Let such agents be content to go forth to the mission field as missionary nurses, not as medical missionaries ; let them, in a quiet, unostentatious way, go about among the homes of the people, searching out the sick and suffering, doing good to all as they have opportunity. Instead of proclaiming themselves " healers of the sick," let them rather disown such a designation—let them frankly acknowledge that they are not, and do not pretend to be doctors, but that they know a little, and may be able in all their common ailments to do them good, and will try to comfort and help them in their greater trials ; let them show their sisters how to make their homes healthier and happier, and let them teach the simple hygienic rules, which they will find everywhere utterly neglected. In such unpretentious but useful work, without raising false expectations, they will find ample scope for the employment of all their energies and talents, and, either single-handed, or, better still, in co-operation with a fully qualified medical missionary, they will do blessed service in the mission field.

In a question of such importance, it is satisfactory to

find, that the views we have expressed are confirmed by the testimony of those whose long experience of professional work in India enables them to speak with authority on this subject, and by that of others who have discovered, by painful experience, the mistake which is made by our Missionary Societies when they send out partially trained ladies as doctors, and impose upon them duties which they are not qualified to discharge.

The well-known Zenana missionary, Miss Beilby, than whom no one, perhaps, has had greater experience as a partially trained medical agent, thus writes—and we ought to state, that the foregoing pages were written before we had the opportunity of knowing Miss Beilby's opinion :—

"Friends of this mission," writes Miss Beilby, "have quoted me as an example of what an unqualified medical missionary can do, but they either forget, or do not know, the circumstances of my case. People see only the outside ; they know nothing of the hours of anxious reading when I ought to have been at rest, and of, at one time, broken health because the burden was too much for me; and also, that when I first went out to India there was not any college or university that gave diplomas or licences to ladies. Whatever I may have done, I should have done better had I been qualified, and should have been free to go on with my work now, instead of having to return to my studies for two or three years. . . . I, with others who have been engaged in Zenana Missions, feel that it is wrong for any woman to call herself a medical missionary, unless she has a full and thorough knowledge of her profession, and has proved she has such, by passing the requisite examination at a college or university. At the same time, I know it is difficult for people who have not been in India to understand this. They hear so much of the dreadful illness and sufferings of the Zenana women, that they think—'Surely an Englishwoman, with two years' good training, could do something to bring relief to those poor sufferers;' but, believe me, it is not 'something,' or 'some relief,' the Zenana lady or her friends want, when the medical missionary is sent for, but it is *everything.* Their own women, *dhais* as they are called, can do something, and one or more of these women will always be sent for before an English lady doctor is called in. . . . When she arrives at the house of her patient, she may be quite sure that, if any ordinary means could do good, she would not have been sent for. I could tell of many cases where, from prolonged suffering, the poor woman has been in such a serious state, that many medical men would have hesitated to undertake such a case alone. It is forgotten, that when a medical lady is in any difficulty she cannot call in another doctor to help her—she must act alone; and although I have always found the medical men where I have worked ready to give me their advice, still how many cases there are in which one needs *more* than advice.

"I was speaking lately, on this subject, to a lady who has been working in India as a medical missionary.

Before she went out, she had been thoroughly trained in
general diseases; and in diseases of women, midwifery,
&c., she was told that nothing more was necessary.  She
is now in London in order to qualify, and this is her
opinion : ' I think it cruel and wicked, for any woman to
go out to India calling herself medical, unless she has
gone through the full course of study, and has a license
or diploma;' and, she adds, ' this is the opinion of all
who know the nature of our work as medical ladies.'   If
Zenana medical missionaries are sent out unqualified,
the missionary work will surely suffer.   The natives are
by no means ignorant of the ways of the world, or of
what is going on in England.   The time was when no
lady could get a license or diploma here, but things are
changed, and none know it better than the native gentlemen of India.   If they send for a lady, calling herself
medical, to attend their female relations, they will expect
to find her qualified, and that she knows her profession
thoroughly. . . . Is there then no sphere for those ladies
who are willing to be trained for two or three years? Yes,
they will be invaluable assistants to the qualified medical
missionaries, if they are willing to work as such ; and in
that case, they should have one year's training as nurses,
and one or two more as assistants. At one time, I thought
it was necessary for the medical missionary herself to be
trained in nursing, but with experience my ideas have
changed, and, while I am thankful for my knowledge of
nursing, I do not think it is necessary for a lady who

intends to qualify, to go through any training in this branch; she should have an assistant to go out with her who understands nursing, and who could train native and East Indian women, as well as help in the medical work. But there is one thing to be guarded against in this, and that is, the unqualified lady should not be sent out two or three years before the qualified one, and when the former has established a missionary work, learned the language, and in all things been first, is told that in the future she must be second, and work under and take her orders from a qualified lady, fresh out from England. People say, 'But if the unqualified person is a Christian, she will do anything that will bring glory to Christ; she will not mind being second where she has been so long first.' It is, in my opinion, doubtful if such an arrangement would bring glory to Christ; one thing I am quite certain of, that however good the unqualified lady was, she would mind very much such a state of things. I would give a word of warning to those who, while thinking all I have said right, might propose to go to India with only a partial knowledge, and then, if they found after some time that they could not get on, return to England and qualify. This is most unwise, for not only is it difficult to recommence studies that have once been put aside, but life and work in India unfit one for hard study. To any one who purposes doing this, I would say most lovingly, as one who has learned from experience, I am sure you will regret such a step all your life."

14

Dr. C. R. Francis, Surgeon-General of H.M. Indian
Army (Retired), and formerly Principal of the Calcutta
Medical College, thus writes on this subject : "A limited
amount of professional knowledge, such as is implied in
missionary students attending lectures and hospital practice
for a year or two, *may* be useful to the missionary in his
solitary tours through secluded regions, or when com-
pletely cut off at his station from all European aid ; but
they who go abroad as *medical missionaries* must be
taught with uncompromising thoroughness.  It must be
remembered that, as civil surgeons are often isolated, the
lady medical missionary may be alone at the mission
station ; and even the presence in it of the civil surgeon
would be no advantage, as he would not be admitted into
the Zenana.  Be the patient ever so ill, she must not see
a man-doctor—death is preferred ; examination of pulse
and tongue through a hole in the 'purda,' or screen,
unsatisfactory at all times, is, in serious sickness when the
patient is prostrate in bed, impossible, and no mere
verbal description of the case would suffice.  Thus
solated, therefore, and cut off from all professional aid,
the lady medical missionary has no one to rely upon but
herself ; and it is to critical cases of this kind that our
ladies may expect to be summoned."  And again, in a
valuable paper on " Medical Women for India," which
appears in "The Journal of the National Indian Association " for February, 1883, Dr. Francis writes : "A word
here on the professional qualifications of the female

medical missionary. Unhappily, there are some—not of any great experience, however—who advocate a limited training with reference to the ordinary illnesses that she will usually be required to treat; granting, for a moment, the force of this (erroneous) argument, what of the extraordinary cases? There may be no one to consult with, and, in her unenviable isolation, the half-educated lady-doctor will then deplore the short-sighted policy of those, who thus sent her imperfectly equipped to a foreign country. By all means prepare intelligent pupils as nurses, with obstetrical qualifications, for India, and let them lay claim to no higher functions; but, in educating the medical missionary who is supposed to be a lady-doctor, do it thoroughly, or not at all. The English public may believe in the apparent *couleur de rose* now, but the results are yet to be seen; and no greater blow could be given to the cause of 'medical women for India,' than the breakdown of those who, each in her own centre, are supposed to represent the professional skill of the West."

We would again state emphatically, that there is a wide field of usefulness, and an urgent demand in the mission field, for well-trained missionary nurses; we cannot send forth too many of such agents: but we would earnestly entreat our ladies' committees not to send them forth as missionary doctors, and we would warn the agents themselves, for their own comfort and usefulness, as well as for the sake of the work, not only not to claim such a designation, but to do all in their power to prevent the natives, among whom they labour, from regarding them in any other light than as nurses.

A few words about the qualifications necessary for the female medical missionary. There is now no longer the excuse, that in this country a fully qualified female medical mission agency cannot be educated and trained. The Henrietta Medical College for Ladies in London provides the necessary instruction, and ladies may now obtain, not only the license of the King and Queen's College of Physicians in Dublin, but, likewise, the medical degree of the London University; for all practical purposes, however, the former is quite sufficient, and may be obtained in less time, and with a less purely scientific course of study, than the London degree. A preliminary examination in general education must be passed before the student can be registered, and allowed to commence her curriculum. This examination includes English, Arithmetic, Algebra, Geometry, Latin, Elementary Mechanics, and either Greek, French, or German. A certificate of having passed the Examination in General Education conducted by certain educational bodies—such as the Universities' Local Examinations (Senior)—is accepted as equivalent to the Medical Preliminary Examinations, provided it includes Latin and Mathematics. The preparation for this honourable service is arduous, and the work itself difficult and anxious; but so far as the supply of fellow-labourers in this increasingly important branch of missionary work is concerned, the Lord knows the need there is for them. Let us then ask them from the Lord, and He will send us brave-hearted, devoted Christian ladies to be educated and trained for this service; let us realize the responsibility that rests upon us, and the deep debt of gratitude we owe for the privileges which we ourselves enjoy; let us give to our sick and suffering heathen sisters the boon we ourselves so highly prize, and which they will hail with gratitude and joy—let us send to the neglected inmates of those Zenanas, the skilled medical aid they so much need, and let us, at the same time, send them the light of the Gospel to enlighten their darkness—to make their dreary homes bright with the sunshine of His presence, and to raise them out of their degradation, to glory, honour, and immortality.

In the closing words of his "Plea for Zenana Medical Missions," Dr. Elmslie writes : " If Florence Nightingale, a thorough English lady—being all that that term implies—left home and friends, and went to Scutari, out of philanthropy, to nurse and doctor England's wounded and dying soldiers, surely other ladies, who have it in their power, should see no insuperable objections or difficulties in giving up home and going to India, to nurse and doctor their needy and suffering sisters *for Christ's sake.* At any rate, India needs female medical missionaries; India will welcome them; India will bless them for their work; and many homes, now dark, will be lighted up through their labours with the knowledge of Him who is the Light of the World.   Surely it is a thing incredible, that among the many Christian daughters of England there are none brave and noble-minded enough to undertake this work, which, of all works, most resembles that of the Great Master Himself, who 'though He was rich, yet for our sakes became poor, that we through His poverty might be made rich,' and of whom it is written, 'Jesus went about all Galilee, teaching in their synagogues, and preaching the Gospel of the Kingdom, and healing all manner of sickness, and all manner of disease among the people.'   'I have given you an ex ample, that ye should do as I have done to you.' "

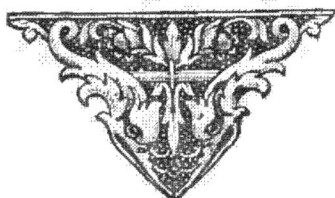

# THE HISTORY AND PROGRESS OF MODERN MEDICAL MISSIONS.

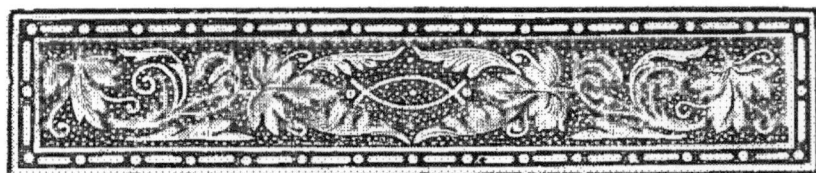

## CHAPTER VIII.

## The History and Progress of Modern Medical Missions. Sketch of the Edinburgh Medical Missionary Society.

THE origin and progress of modern medical missions are closely identified with the history of the Edinburgh Medical Missionary Society ; for although upwards of sixty years ago Mr. Douglas of Cavers, in his " Hints on Missions," pointed out the advantages likely to be derived from the employment of this agency, it was not till nearly twenty years after that useful little work was published, that the attention of the friends of missions in this country was directed to the subject.

In 1841, the Rev. Peter Parker, M.D., a medical missionary from America, who had laboured for many years, and with much success in China, passed through Edinburgh on his way to the United States. During his short visit to Edinburgh, he was the guest of the late Dr. Abercrombie, who was so greatly interested in the intelligence he received from him, especially with his experience of the value of the healing art as a pioneer to missionary effort, that he invited to his house a few friends, to hear Dr. Parker's account of his work, and to consider the propriety of forming an association in Edinburgh, for the purpose of promoting medical missions.

As the result of the interest thus awakened, a public meeting was held on 30th November of the same year, when the following resolution was adopted and the Society formed : "That this meeting, being deeply sensible of the beneficial results which may be expected to arise from the labours of Christian medical men co-operating with missionaries in various parts of the world, thus giving intelligent proofs of the nature and practical operation of the spirit of love which, as the fruit of our holy religion, we desire to see diffused amongst all nations, resolve to promote this object, and to follow the leadings of Providence, by encouraging in every possible way the settlement of Christian medical men in foreign countries, and that, for this purpose, a Society be formed, under the name of the 'Edinburgh Association for Sending Medical Aid to Foreign Countries.'" It was at the same time resolved, that "The objects of the Association shall be, to circulate information on the subject, to endeavour to originate and aid such kindred institutions as may be formed to prosecute the same work, and to render assistance at missionary stations to as many professional agents as the funds placed at its disposal may admit."

Dr. Abercrombie was chosen President, and, till his death in November, 1844, he took the warmest interest in the operations of the Society. Others there were, of world-wide reputation, whose names are identified with its origin. The Rev. Dr. Thomas Chalmers and Professor Alison were elected Vice-Presidents at the inaugural meeting. Dr. James Begbie, Professor Sir George Ballingall, Dr. William Beilby (who succeeded Dr. Abercrombie as President), Professor Syme, Dr. John Coldstream, Mr. Joseph Bell, Dr. Omond, Dr. Handyside—all well-known and honoured names—are found among the first list of Directors. Two only of the original Directors are still spared (1886) to take part in the management of the Society, namely, the respected President, Mr. William Brown, F.R.C.S.E., and the Rev. G. D. Cullen, M.A., Vice-President.

On November 28, 1843, the second annual meeting was held, when it was resolved that "henceforth the Association shall be designated 'The Edinburgh Medical Missionary Society.'" The income of the Society during the first year of its existence amounted to only £114, and at the close of its first decade the annual income had never exceeded £300. Till 1851, the funds of the Society were mainly expended in diffusing medical missionary information. Lectures on the subject of

Medical Missions were delivered by several of the Directors, and afterwards published and widely circulated; prizes were offered for the best essays on this subject, and every available opportunity taken to advocate the claims of this new and interesting department of missionary service. From time to time, grants of money for the purchase of medicines and instruments were made to the few medical missionaries then at work in the foreign field.

From a list of Protestant Medical Missionaries, printed as an appendix to the Tenth Annual Report of the Society, we find that previous to 1841, only three such agents from this country were engaged in this work, namely, Dr. Lockhart at Shanghai, Dr. Hobson at Hongkong, and afterwards at Canton, both in connection with the London Missionary Society; and Dr. Kalley, who, unconnected with any society, went out to Madeira in 1837. At the close of 1852, there were thirteen European medical missionaries employed in India, China, and elsewhere, as the agents of the various missionary societies; one of these, Dr. Wallace, being supported by the Edinburgh Medical Missionary Society as a missionary to the Roman Catholics in Ireland.

In reviewing the first ten years of the Society's history, the Report for 1852 thus refers to the work accomplished, and to the future prospects of the cause : " We feel satisfied that the subject of Medical Missions is gradually becoming more familiar to the public mind, that there is a growing interest in its favour, and that, at no distant period, its importance will be universally seen and acknowledged. Let us look upon the last ten years as the vernal period of the Society, during which we have been mainly occupied in preparing the soil and scattering the seed ; and let us anticipate a season—not far distant, we trust—when the silent and unseen germinating process, which is now advancing, will declare itself by a sudden growth of fresh and vigorous manifestation ; and for this we must look upwards in faith to Him on whose rain and sunshine the spiritual no less than the natural husbandry exclusively depends."

As the results of medical missionary effort became more widely know, the demand for this form of agency increased, and the various Societies naturally looked to the Edinburgh Medical Missionary Society for the supply of men ready for the work. Early in the second decade of the Society's history, therefore, the necessity arose of embracing, as part of its aims and objects, the helping forward of suitable young men, who, having given evidence that they were impelled by the constraining influence of the love of Christ, had resolved to dedicate themselves to His service as medical missionaries. This important, and now extensive, department of the Society's work was entered upon by the Directors with certainly very humble pretentions, as indicated by the following *minute*, recorded in June, 1851, which takes us back to the origin of the Society's Training Institution : "The Committee resolved to devote part of the funds at their

disposal to the supplying of one or more students with
the means of prosecuting their professional education,
in order to enable them to prepare for entering upon
medical missionary service."

For several years the aid rendered to students was
merely pecuniary. The Directors, indeed, took a warm
interest in those they were helping forward, and endeavoured by every means in their power to foster in
them the missionary spirit; but so far as providing opportunities for training them for the work was concerned,
their connection with the Society at this early stage conferred upon the students no special advantage. In a
remarkable way, however, this want was, in God's providence, ere long supplied.

On October 30, 1848; Dr. Handyside—whose name
has already been mentioned as one of the first Directors,
and who, till his death, which took place early in 1881,
was one of the Society's truest and most devoted friends—
received a note from the Rev. P. McMenamy, then a
missionary to the Irish in Edinburgh, asking him if he
would kindly undertake to visit professionally some of
his sick poor. In the spirit of true Christian philanthropy Dr. Handyside at once consented, and henceforth, wherever there were sick and suffering Irish, there,
along with their missionary, the doctor was to be found.
It was not long till Dr. Handyside discovered, that the
kind and successful treatment of the wounded and
diseased body, opened a way for the application of the

"balm of Gilead" to the sin-stricken soul; and, revolving in his mind how best to turn to account the influence thus acquired, the idea suggested itself of establishing a medical mission dispensary. In dependence on that blessing from the Lord which is promised to him "that considereth the poor," Dr. Handyside resolved to make the experiment, and on November 25, 1853, he opened the "Main Point Mission Dispensary;" and as this was the first *Home* Medical Mission in Great Britain, and the origin of the Society's Training Institution, the following brief extract from the First Annual Report is interesting, as showing the principle upon which it was founded, and the spirit in which the work was carried on : "The Saviour, when on earth, manifested the tenderest pity for the afflicted, but while He was ever ready to afford them bodily relief, He never failed at the same time to minister to their spiritual wants. In this 'He hath left us an example that we should follow His steps.' The Gospel is the discovery of the grace of God to man, and the unfeigned belief of it will produce a disposition to 'do good unto all men as we have opportunity.' It is in accordance alike with Scripture and reason that we should employ such an agency; but, unless the blessing and help of God are implored, and the grace so freely bestowed is received, human effort can never be successful in alleviating the distress, enlightening the mind, and elevating the character of those among whom we labour."

We have here set forth, at the very inauguration of Home Medical Missions, the true principle and grand aim of the enterprise. Some there were, at this early stage, who, ignorant of the mode of carrying on the work, had their misgivings about it, and, for no well-defined reason, refused their sympathy and support; others regarded the evangelistic element either, as taking an unfair advantage to proselytize, or, as a veiled attempt to force religion upon the poor patient. Some objected to the physician undertaking duties which, in their opinion, belonged only to the minister of religion or to the missionary; while not a few, fully recognizing the value of the agency, and impressed with the force of the Divine precept and example, rallied round Dr. Handyside, and cordially co-operated with him; and the hopes of those early friends of the cause were not disappointed.

Dr. Handyside, from the first, associated with himself the young men preparing for medical missionary service in connection with the Society, and as they thus had opportunities, day by day, of addressing the patients assembled in the waiting-room, and of speaking a word in season at the bedside of the afflicted, while at the same time, under Dr. Handyside's guidance, they ministered to their bodily ailments, they felt that, in view of the work to which they were looking forward, the privileges they enjoyed in connection with the "Main Point Mission Dispensary" were of inestimable value.

In 1858, the attendance of patients had so largely

increased, that it was found absolutely necessary to
secure more suitable and commodious premises.    In
the providence of God, the way was opened for obtaining excellent accommodation in the best locality in the
city for planting such a mission.    One day, in the spring
of 1858, as Dr. Handyside passed along the Cowgate
on one of his errands of mercy, he observed a board
with "To Let" upon it, above the door of No. 39,
which was till then one of the numerous whisky shops
in that long, narrow street.    This, he thought, is like
the place we are looking out for, and it is certainly
in the right locality.    He went in, looked round the
premises, and saw at once that, with a little outlay, they
could be made most suitable.    He found that the
spirit dealer had a lease of the shop for a considerable
time, but that he was willing to accept a reasonable
offer for the remainder of the lease, and at once to give
over the premises.    Within a few days, satisfactory
terms were agreed upon, and at Whitsunday, 1858, the
" old whisky shop," 39, Cowgate, was transformed into
a Medical Mission Dispensary.

Soon after the removal of the "Main Point Mission
Dispensary" to the Cowgate, the students then in connection with the Society presented a memorial to the
Directors, in which they expressed their appreciation of
the many and great privileges which they enjoyed under
Dr. Handyside, and testified to the fact, that such an
institution as the " Cowgate Mission Dispensary " is the

15

best apprentice school for the medical missionary student. They urged, too, the importance of the Directors having opportunities of knowing what progress their students were making in their studies, as well as of training them, and thereby testing their fitness for missionary work; and concluded by stating their conviction, that the amalgamation of the Cowgate Dispensary with the Edinburgh Medical Missionary Society would be a union fraught with rich results.

Dr. Handyside warmly supported the memorial, and on the 18th November, 1861, the "Cowgate Mission Dispensary" became the "Edinburgh Medical Missionary Society's Training Institution"—a union which has been greatly blessed to the furtherance of the cause of medical missions, and which makes specially memorable, this second decade of the Society's history.

In other respects, the Society during this period made gradual but decided progress. It commenced, along with the Free Church of Scotland, a medical mission in Madras, and, conjointly with the London Missionary Society, it supported for four years a medical missionary at Mirzapore. It established a medical mission in Ireland, and supported the medical missionary there for six years. During the period under review, several well-known medical missionaries were helped forward by the Society, in their preparation for the work, among whom were Mr. David Paterson, F.R.C.S.E., the Society's first student, and for more

than ten years its devoted agent at Madras; Dr. Wong
Fun of Canton, the first Chinese graduate of a European
University, and for many years the colleague of the
veteran medical missionary, Dr. Hobson; Dr. James
Henderson of Shanghai, whose memoir every young
man should read, and Dr. James Bell of Amoy, all of
whom now rest from their labours.   Dr. Colin Valentine, Superintendent of the Agra Medical Missionary
Training Institution, Dr. Vartan of Nazareth, and the
writer, all students of the Society during the same period,
are still spared for service in the medical mission field.
By the publication of an " Occasional Paper," and by
public meetings and lectures, much was done by the
Society during these years to promote an interest in the
cause, and its income rose from £350 in 1852, to
£1250 in 1862.

Under the superintendence of Mr. W. Burns Thomson, F.R.C.S.E., who, while agent of the Society from
1860 till 1870, laboured with much success and enthusiasm to promote the cause of medical missions,
the training institution soon became, not only thoroughly
efficient, but likewise, a powerful and much blessed local
benevolent and evangelistic agency.   In the annual
report of the Society for 1865, the following reference
is made to the progress of the work : " A general
retrospect of the period since the amalgamation of the
Dispensary with the Society, calls for thankfulness and
praise; for it is known by those mainly engaged in the

work, that many of the lowest and most degraded of the population resorting thither, have not only heard the gracious offer of the Gospel, but have become partakers of the salvation which is in Christ Jesus. Not a few, believed to be now in glory, gave testimony before their departure that they were born again; and a goodly number still living regard the Superintendent and his fellow-workers as their fathers in Christ. Year by year, the value of the institution as a training school for missionaries is becoming more and more apparent; and it would be difficult, we imagine, to find a band of more devoted and accomplished young men than those who have already issued from its walls."

Ere long, it was found necessary to provide increased accommodation, and a lease was obtained of the adjoining premises, the lower part of which was converted into a consulting-room, laboratory, and waiting-room, and the upper part comfortably furnished as a residence for the Superintendent and the students; a further step was thus taken in the development of this important department of the Society's work.

In 1863, the Society sustained a heavy loss in the death of Dr. John Coldstream, who had been associated with Mr. Benjamin Bell, F.R.C.S.E., as Secretary almost from its commencement. Dr. Coldstream's name was, up till this period, intimately identified with the entire history of the institution; and to his unwearied devotion, wise counsel, and sanctified enthusiasm for the cause of medical missions, much of the success which had hitherto attended the Society's operations may be traced. Several medical missionaries, and among them the writer, trace much of the interest which they have been led to take in this department of missionary work to their intercourse with Dr. Coldstream. A medical missionary scholarship, of the annual value of £25, has been founded, as a memorial of that " beloved physician " and earnest promoter of the cause.

In the following year (1864), the Society sustained another heavy loss in the death of Professor Miller, one of its Vice-Presidents, a warm friend and eloquent advocate of medical missions. His eminent service to the Society as an expounder of its principles, the deep interest he ever manifested in all departments of its work, and especially, as convener of the Students' Aid Committee, his affectionate and earnest solicitude for the welfare of the students, and withal, his unostentatious zeal for the promotion of the Redeemer's cause, invested him with an influence which carried with it an almost irresistible charm. The last public duty he discharged was to lecture on behalf of the Society, and the burden of his address, on that occasion, was the value of the Cowgate institution as a training school for medical missionaries, and the important relation it sustains to medical mission work abroad. It was one of the purposes of his life—an object for which he prayed, and pleaded, and worked—to get this central institution efficiently equipped, and put into thorough working order, believing that thus, the Society would best fulfil its mission at home, and be able to meet the ever-increasing demands of the foreign field.

Soon after the death of Professor Miller, his many friends and admirers resolved to raise a memorial fund, in order, in some way, to associate his name with the work of the training institution which he loved so well. Upwards of £2000 was soon raised, and with this sum the Committee purchased, and furnished, the convenient and commodious house, 56, George Square, now known as the "Miller Memorial Medical Mission House," and handed it over to the Society, as a residence for the Superintendent and the students.   In God's providence, another, and much felt, want was thus supplied; for although " 39, Cowgate" was the locality, of all others, best suited for carrying on the practical work of the training institution, still, the premises, as they then existed, were far from being a desirable residence for the workers.

While the Cowgate Dispensary was thus gradually developing into an institution of goodly proportions, the operations of the Society were at the same time branching out, and making their influence felt in other directions. From time to time, the Superintendent and those of the Directors best acquainted with the work, visited the larger towns and cities, as deputations, to plead the cause of the Society ; and as the success of the medical mission work carried on in the Cowgate thus became better known, interest was awakened, and ere very long, Medical Mission Dispensaries were opened in Glasgow, Aberdeen, Liverpool, London, Manchester, and other centres, so that now, in many places we find flourishing mission dispensaries, and wherever these have been established they are recognized as powerful auxiliaries to home mission work.

Early in 1870, Mr. W. Burns Thomson resigned his connection with the Society, and was succeeded by Mr. David Paterson, F.R.C.S.E., whose fifteen years of devoted and successful service, as the Society's agent at Madras, eminently qualified him for the position he was called to occupy at the head of the training institution ; but the Master had nobler service for him in a holier sphere.    After only four brief months of home work as Superintendent, Mr. Paterson died on February 14, 1871.

Shortly before the death of Mr. Paterson, the Rev. John Lowe, F.R.C.S.E., medical missionary in connection with the London Missionary Society in Travancore, then at home on furlough on account of the failure of his wife's health, received a very decided medical opinion, that it would be at the risk of her life should Mrs. Lowe again return to India.    Under these circumstances, towards the end of January, Mr. Lowe resigned his connection with the London Missionary Society, and on the death of Mr. Paterson the Directors had their thoughts at once directed to him.    His connection as a student with the Cowgate Dispensary from its commencement, his eight years' experience of medical missionary work in India, the providential circumstances which, just then, had left him no alternative but to give up all thought of resuming his work in Travancore, the urgent claims of the Society, the unanimous invitation of its Directors, and the advice of friends, all clearly indicated the path of duty.    Mr. Lowe accepted the appointment, and on the 1st of March, 1871, entered upon his duties as Superintendent of the Society's Training Institution.

The Report of the Society for the year 1870 closes with these words : "Some still remember the small beginning of our enterprise, and the difficulties of every kind which beset our inexperienced footsteps, and which, one by one, have been overcome, until the modest aid-giving Committee with which we began has expanded by an unlooked-for growth, and without any preconceived plan of ours, into an institution of goodly and still increasing dimensions. Your Directors, impressed by these things, are more convinced than ever that the Lord is favouring the work, and that no step can be safely taken apart from His guidance, who has all along been leading us by a way we knew not—opening it here, closing it there ; disappointing cherished hopes to-day, and to-morrow, crowning them with unlooked-for favour and success !    Let us then be more earnest in prayer as regards the future.    *Without* God's Holy Spirit we are absolutely helpless, alike as individuals and as a society ; *with* His indwelling presence and help, nothing is too great to be achieved—a lesson which, again and again, has been taught us during the past quarter of a century."

In 1861 the income of the Society was £590; in 1871 it amounted to £1314.

The last decade of the Society's history (1871–81) is, however, the period during which it has made the greatest progress. One or two facts will illustrate this. In 1871 there were only seven students preparing for medical missionary work under the auspices of the Society; in 1881 there were sixteen. There are at present upwards of one hundred and seventy qualified medical missionaries in active service at home and abroad—of these only thirty were in the field previous to 1871. As already stated, the income of the Society in 1871 was £1314, in 1881 it amounted to £5506; while, during the decade, upwards of £15,000 were raised for special objects, independently of the Society's general income. The erection of the new and commodious premises, in which the work is now carried on, marks the beginning of a new era in the history of the Society.

A few years ago the "old whisky shop," with its dingy surroundings, was swept away, and on its site there now stands the "Livingstone Memorial Medical Missionary Training Institution," a most fitting national expression of admiration of the character, and sympathy with the life-work, of the great African explorer whose name it bears, himself a medical missionary, and for nearly twenty years a corresponding member of the Edinburgh Medical Missionary Society. A site might have been chosen, indeed one was actually secured, which would have given the Institution a prominence which in the Cowgate it cannot have; but, like Livingstone himself, who lived, laboured, and died for the reclamation of the wastes of heathenism, this Memorial Missionary Institute is most appropriately planted, in the very midst of the moral and spiritual wastes of our home heathenism, for the alleviation of human suffering and the salvation of the lost, and, at the same time, for the training of young missionaries who shall follow in the footsteps of Livingstone—or, rather, in the footsteps of His and their great Master—and who shall go forth with healing in the one hand for the afflicted body, and in the other "the balm of Gilead" for the sin-sick soul.

The memorial-stone of the "Livingstone Memorial" was laid by the late Rev. Robert Moffat, D.D., on June 9, 1877, in the presence of a large number of spectators, the late Sir John McNeill, G.C.B., presiding. In the course of his address, Sir John congratulated the company on the presence in their midst, of the one man living whom, on such an occasion they would most desire to see. He referred to Dr. Moffat, who was the representative of the great missionary explorer in whose honour they were met. Of the life and labours of Dr. Livingstone he would not attempt to speak. They well knew his devotion, his piety, his courage, his indomitable perseverance even unto death. They knew the cause for which he laboured—that he was the pioneer of Christianity and of civilization in the heart of Africa—that it was to him they owed the knowledge that Central Africa, instead of being a barren unpeopled waste, was a country densely populated, to whose people he was the first to carry the tidings of hope. He was sure none of them would ever regret having taken part in this interesting ceremony, but rather, in days to come, would they remember with pleasure the share they had taken in promoting an institution which, in its operations, embodied most nearly an approach to our Saviour's example.

Mr. Lowe, Superintendent of the Training Institution, after giving a brief historical sketch of the work, said : "In the heart of down-trodden and oppressed Africa, Livingstone's faithful servants built him a hut in which to die ; in the heart of this sin-blighted moral waste, we are building him a house in which he, being dead, shall yet speak. Early in the morning of the 1st of May 1873, Dr. Livingstone was found within that rude hut, kneeling by the side of his bed—his body stretched forward—his head buried in his hands upon the pillow. For a minute his servants watched him—he did not stir—there was no sign of breathing ; then one of them, Matthew, advanced softly and placed his hand to his cheek; it was sufficient— life had been extinct some time, and the body was almost cold—Livingstone was dead ! In view of the interesting ceremony we are now to witness, it is profitable thus to recall the last moments of the great and good man, whose name and memory we desire to honour. Livingstone died in the attitude of prayer—his whole life was a prayer, and, as all prayer should be, practical, fulfilling itself. And what is the noble effort of the Free Church at Livingstonia? and that of the Established Church of Scotland at Blantyre? and what the missions that are being founded by Dr. Smith, our former resident here, and his devoted associates, in connection with the Church Missionary Society on the shores of the Victoria Nyanza? and that by the London Missionary Society at Ujiji on Lake Tanganyika? and that by the Universities' Mission on the Shiré? and what is the noble enterprise of our friends, the brothers Moir? and what is this Memorial Training Institution, from whence, we trust and pray, many earnest, devoted, medical missionaries will go forth to carry the blessings of Christianity and civilization to Africa and other heathen lands? What are all these grand enterprises but the direct answer to Livingstone's life-long prayer—the last feeble utterances of which were wafted to heaven, as he knelt over his bed in that lonely hut, and gently breathed his spirit home to God? The lesson taught by all these grand undertakings, connected as they are with the life and death of Livingstone, is, "Be not weary in well doing, for in due season ye shall reap if ye faint not."

> " Work in the wild waste places,
>   Though none thy love may own ;

God guides the down of the thistle
The wandering wind hath sown.
Will Jesus chide thy weakness,
Or call thy labour vain ?
The word that for Him thou bearest
Will return to Him again
On, with thy heart in heaven !
Thy strength the Master's might !
Till the wild waste places blossom
In the warmth of a Saviour's light."

Mr. Lowe then presented Dr. Moffat with a silver trowel, the gift of the Directors, expressing the hope that he might long be spared to keep it in his possession as a memento of this interesting ceremony, and that it might be handed down to generations of those bearing the honoured name of Livingstone !

The hymn "Tell it out among the heathen" was sung by the children of the Children's Church connected with the Mission, and Dr. Moffat then laid the memorial-stone, a hermetically sealed bottle having been placed in the cavity containing photographs of Dr. Livingstone and of his venerable father-in-law, Dr. Moffat; also copies of the Edinburgh newspapers of that day, and of the *Quarterly Paper* of the Edinburgh Medical Missionary Society. On the front of the stone the following inscription is cut : " LIVINGSTONE MEDICAL MISSIONARY MEMORIAL. THE REV. ROBERT MOFFAT, D.D., LAID THIS STONE, JUNE 9th, 1877.

After prayer by the Rev. Dr. Murray Mitchell, Dr. Moffat said he could not exaggerate the pleasure he felt on the present occasion, but it was impossible for him to stand there and witness what he had just seen, and hear what he had heard, without peculiar emotion. He knew the man whose name was to be kept in remembrance by this building, and he could not have other than a heart overflowing with gratitude, in witnessing the commencement of an undertaking, intended for the training of those who were to devote themselves to the glorious purpose for which he spent his life, and in the interests of which he died! It was scarcely necessary for him to say more in reference to the character of the Institution than that which had been so well said already. It was indeed a noble institution, and no word from him was required to commend it to public attention. Wherever medical missionaries had gone, they had left their mark, and they had been greatly honoured in their labours. He had had innumerable opportunities of witnessing the value of medical missionary work. He had often said, and he said it again, that a missionary was a good thing—and any one who knew the work they did must say so ; but a *medical* missionary was a missionary and a half, or rather, he should say, a double missionary ! It was impossible to estimate the value of a missionary going out with a thorough knowledge of medicine and surgery. When he went out, there was no such agency thought of by the Missionary Societies. He knew little about medicine, and the missionaries who accompanied him knew still less. He did know a little, for when he was a boy he fell in with a packman with a few books for sale, and amongst them, he happened to select "Buchan's Domestic Medicine," which seemed to imply that something was to follow. In after life he found it necessary to add to his medical library, and to enlarge his knowledge of medicine, and was able, in some way or other, to doctor the people; and the more experience he had in that direction, the more useful and successful were his services. He would just mention, in reference to their dear departed friend, Dr. Livingstone, that he (Dr. Moffat) had innumerable opportunities of witnessing the influence he gained over the natives, by the successful use of his knowledge of medicine and surgery. He had himself often seen the willingness he showed, the sacrifices he made, and how often he exposed himself to danger, in order to alleviate suffering or save life. He had left a bright name behind him, and it would be well remembered by, and most appropriately associated with, this building; and so long as he was able to appeal on behalf of missions, he wouldplead for this Institution, and for the Edinburgh Medical Missionary Society.

Mr. Brown, F.R.C.S.E. President of the Society, expressed to Sir John McNeill the thanks of the directors and friends for his kindness in presiding, and Mr. Bell, F.R.C.S.E., Secretary of the Society, thanked Dr. Moffat. The interesting proceedings were brought to a close by the children singing, "How beautiful upon the mountains."

In the middle of December, in the same year, a Bazaar was held in the Music Hall, Edinburgh, under the patronage of H.R.II. The Princess Louise, in order to complete the sum required for the erection and equipment of the new Institution. The sum realized by this bazaar, and a more private supplementary sale held afterwards, was nearly £5000. The expenses, amounting only to £388, were more than met by the entrance money. The bazaar, a pleasant memory to all who took any part in it, was a great success. It was free from many of the evils which are so often attendant on this method of raising money for good objects. No raffling was allowed, while many who visited the bazaar remarked on the high tone which pervaded it. It was a Christian enterprise carried on in a truly Christian spirit.

On the 25th of January, 1878, the Livingstone Memorial Medical Missionary Training Institution was inaugurated by a dedication service; while, on the following evening, a social entertainment was given in the waiting-room, to the poor people resident in the neighbourhood.

The Memorial, with its furnishings, cost nearly £10,000, and before the building was finished the required amount had been fully provided. The locality is rich in historical associations; especially do these cluster round the Magdalen Chapel, which has descended to us, in wonderful preservation, from Pre-Reformation times. This ecclesiastical relic belongs to the Protestant Institute, but, by special arrangement, it is incorporated with, and

forms part of, the Livingstone Memorial Training Institution, the front elevation of which corresponds with that
of the old Magdalen, which has been beautifully restored,
both externally and internally, and is now utilized for
carrying on the evangelistic services in connection with
the Mission. In this antique chapel the arms of the
founder, Michael Macquhan, are seen on the old
stained-glass window, side by side with those of Mary of
Guise. Hence the light of Divine truth radiated when
Scotland separated from Rome ; and here, in 1578, the
first General Assembly of the Church of Scotland was
held—Mr. Andrew Melville moderator. Round the
walls are eighty-eight beautifully carved oak panels,
commemorative of the gifts to "ye crosse house" of
many worthies long since departed. In the south-east
corner is the tomb of "Dame Macquhan, ane honoribil
woman, and decessist ye iii of December, A.D. 1553;"
and here, too, is the old table upon which was laid the
body of the martyred Duke of Argyll, after his execution
in the Grass-market in 1665, with other interesting relics
well worthy the inspection of the antiquary.

It is not a little curious to discover, by the following
advertisement, which appears in the *Scots Postman* of
September 21st, 1710, that, fully one hundred and
seventy years ago, the house adjoining the Magdalen
Chapel, on the site of which now stands the Livingstone
Memorial Medical Mission Training Institution, was
used as a dispensary :—" In the Hammer-mens-land at

the Magdalen Chapel, near the head of the Cowgate, lives Anthony Parsons, who, in his travels, above thirty years in this and other countries, has attained to the method of curing many diseases incident to men, women, and children—more especially those of the eyes; and according to the best of his knowledge, lets the patient know if curable or not."

The Memorial Institute in outward appearance is solid, simple, and unpretending; while internally, it is commodious, and well adapted for all the purposes it is intended to serve. The ground-floor contains the janitor's residence, the laboratory, consulting-room, vaccination or class-room, and a waiting-room comfortably seated for one hundred and fifty. Here, there has been some slight indulgence in ornamentation, which no one will grudge in a place where the depressed and suffering daily congregate. The east end of the room is adorned with a beautiful stained-glass window, the gift of several hundreds of the poor patients themselves; the centre of the window represents our Lord healing the sick—on the one side are the words, "Himself took our infirmities," and on the other, "and bare our sicknesses." On the second floor, are the resident physician's parlour, the matron's parlour and bed-room, the kitchen, servants' room, and dining-hall, in which there is a very handsome marble bust of Dr. Livingstone, and an oil painting of Dr. Moffat. The third floor is occupied by the library, and bed-room parlours of the students.

The wide-spread and successful efforts made to raise the funds necessary for the erection of the Livingstone Memorial, gave a great impulse to the cause of medical missions. Many then learned, for the first time, that such an organization existed, and that such a Christ-like work was carried on, and these have ever since been liberal supporters of the Society.

Since 1872, upwards of forty students have been educated and trained for their work in the Institution. Legally qualified medical missionaries have been supplied by this Society, to the Church Missionary Society, the London Missionary Society, the Established Church of Scotland, the Free Church, United Presbyterian, English Presbyterian, Irish Presbyterian, Scottish Episcopal, Baptist, and Methodist New Connexion Missionary Societies; to the China Inland Mission, the American Board of Commissioners for Foreign Missions, the American Methodist Missionary Society, as well as to several Home Medical Missions. The students belong to the various evangelical denominations, and are drawn from all parts of the United Kingdom, and from other countries. The Society, in its constitution, and in its practical operations, provides a platform upon which all, of whatever name or denomination, who love the Lord Jesus Christ, and whose prayer is "Thy kingdom come," may join hand in hand in a holy alliance for the advancement of His dominion, which "shall extend from sea to sea, and from the river unto the ends of the earth."

We must not omit to mention that the Edinburgh Medical Missionary Society has established several flourishing medical missions in the foreign field. Reference has already been made to two of these missions, namely, the Nazareth Medical Mission, and the Medical Mission at Madras; the latter, however, has been lately transferred to the Free Church of Scotland. In 1874, the Society established a most successful medical mission at Niigata, Japan, which has just been transferred to the American Board of Commissioners for Foreign Missions; and more recently, it has sent forth Dr. Mackinnon to commence medical mission work in Damascus. It assisted Miss de Broen in the inauguration of the Belleville Medical Mission in Paris, and paid the salary of the medical missionary there for the first two years; while within the last few years, it has remitted upwards of £2000, in grants for the purchase of medicines, instruments, &c., to medical missionaries labouring in India, China, Africa, Turkey, Syria, Egypt, Rome, and in other lands and islands of the sea.

These are a few outstanding indications of the Divine blessing resting upon the work of the Society, and upon the cause, with the progress of which it has been so closely identified during the past forty-four years; but there are other indications which we cannot tabulate, and which inspire us with still greater hopefulness than even the encouraging facts to which we have referred. We allude to the increasing appreciation of this form of agency, and to the intelligent interest which has been awakened in the work. Apologetic pleading on behalf of medical missions is not now called for; the work approves itself to every true-hearted Christian, and the objections to medical missions which were rife five and twenty years ago, are now never even heard. It was difficult formerly to obtain appointments for the medical missionary students as they finished their course of preparation ; now the demand is greater than the supply. As already stated, there are now, in active service, at home and abroad, upwards of one hundred and seventy qualified medical missionaries, of whom not more than thirty were in the field in 1870; while, from time to time, almost every missionary periodical tells the story of medical missionary triumphs in all parts of the world.

In closing their last Annual Report, the Directors of the Edinburgh Medical Missionary Society say : " We would ask all interested in the cause of medical missions to join with us in humble and hearty thanksgiving to God, for the large measure of success and blessing which He hath so graciously vouchsafed upon all departments of the Society's work. Financially, and otherwise, the past year has been perhaps the most prosperous in our history. Large demands have been made upon our resources, both for home and foreign work, but these demands have been created by the very fulness of the Divine blessing which has rested upon the Society's operations ; and it is very pleasing to observe that, in a corresponding measure, the Lord hath graciously inclined the hearts of His people to send liberal help. We must not, however, rest content with our present position. The experience of the past, the ever increasing interest in the work, the vantage ground which, as a Society, we occupy, the resources which, when needed, have always been provided—in short, God's providential dealings with us, all conspire to urge us forward ; we would hear His voice in all, saying to us, ' Enlarge the place of thy tent, and stretch forth the curtains of thine habitations ; spare not, lengthen thy cords, and strengthen thy stakes, for thou shalt break forth on the right hand, and on the left.' "

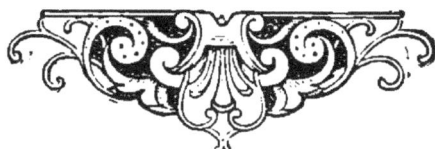

# HOME MEDICAL MISSIONS; THEIR PLACE, METHOD, AND POWER.

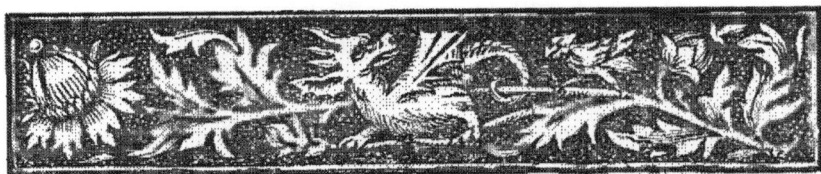

## CHAPTER IX.

### Home Medical Missions; their place, method, and power.

WHILE our chief object is to illustrate the value of medical missions, and to promote the more general employment of this agency as an auxiliary to missionary work abroad, yet the treatment of our subject would be incomplete without some reference to medical mission work at home.

In this department, we again find the Edinburgh Medical Missionary Society taking the lead. The first Home medical mission, however, although established and supported by that society, was not located in Edinburgh, but in Ireland. In 1848, the late Rev. Dr. Carlile, of Parsonstown, King's County, Ireland, wrote a very interesting letter to the Directors of the Edinburgh Medical Missionary Society, stating, in a very strong and effective manner, the claims of Ireland as a field for medical missionary effort, and requesting them, if possible, to send him a medical coadjutor to act as a missionary at Birr, where an active evangelistic mission had just been established by the Irish Presbyterian Church. " I have for many years thought," wrote Dr. Carlile, "that Ireland should be treated just like any other mission field, and that it required even more delicacy and energy of treatment than almost any other; and so far back as 1825, I printed an appeal in which I urged, among other measures, the employment of missionary physicians. My residence in the heart of Ireland for eight years, has confirmed my opinion as to the need of such an agency, and has made me exceedingly anxious that at least the experiment should be made."

China was the field which the Directors had intended to occupy so soon as they were in a position to support an agent of their own, and, conscious of their dependence on the Divine blessing, they resolved to hold a monthly prayer-meeting to implore God's help and guidance in reference to this special matter. These meetings, the first of which was held in April, 1848, were most precious and profitable seasons to all who were privileged to take part in them. At the second meeting, Dr. Carlile's letter was read, and was received as a direct answer to prayer. After mature consideration, the Directors resolved to respond to Dr. Carlile's request, and, should a suitable agent be found, to support a medical missionary at Birr; but meanwhile, they determined to relax none of their efforts on behalf of China. The Committee frequently met for prayer that some one qualified for the work might offer his services as a medical missionary to Ireland. They did not wait long, for early in August the same year, Dr. Alexander W. Wallace, a young graduate of Edinburgh University, applied for the appointment, and having produced most satisfactory testimonials as to his qualifications, both medical and missionary, he was forthwith appointed. Writing to the Committee, a few months after Dr. Wallace had entered upon his duties at Birr, Dr. Carlile expressed his great satisfaction with the result of the "experiment," as he termed it. "It is," he says, "with much thankfulness, that I have to own that God appears peculiarly to smile on the experiment which you have made in sending us a medical missionary. I bless God that I was led, I trust by His Spirit, to suggest the measure to your Society, and that you were led, I trust by the same Spirit, to comply with the request I then made, and that He provided for you one so well qualified in every way as Dr. Wallace. He is rapidly gaining the confidence of the people; his hands are quite full of work, and several, who were well known to us as our most bigoted and violent opponents, have been consulting him. He is everything that my fondest hopes could desire—zealous in his profession, and equally so for the glory of God."

In his dispensary, and in visiting patients at their own homes, while he successfully discharged his duties as a

physician, Dr. Wallace availed himself most assiduously
of every opportunity to commend to his patients the truth
as it is in Jesus, and many were led to acknowledge
themselves indebted to him, as the instrument in leading
them to the Saviour, the source of all true peace.   He
was, ere long, welcomed in many quarters, where formerly
he had been abused, stoned, and driven from the doors.
Two years after he had settled at Birr, Dr. Carlile wrote :
" We may now say that all opposition to the doctor has
ceased.    We are every day hearing of people who
formerly were most violent in their opposition giving way
—some of them consulting him, and others cordially
acknowledging the value of his services ; and it is encouraging to be able to add, that this change has taken
place in the mind of the people simultaneously with his
more openly and decidedly prosecuting the higher object
of his mission.   As the result of his work, I believe a
great change is silently and gradually passing over the
community here."

Dr. Wallace carried on his work at Birr, as the agent
of the Society, till 1855, when the passing of the Medical
Relief Bill limited, to a great extent, his usefulness ; and
this circumstance, along with the fact, that extensive
emigration from the locality had entirely changed the
character of the district, as a sphere for medical missionary
work, led the Directors to relinquish the mission at Birr,
and to concentrate their efforts on some part of the
foreign field.

Let us hope, that this brief allusion to the *first* Home Medical Mission may awaken, in the minds of those interested in Irish evangelization, a desire to promote medical mission work among the poor of that unhappy and distracted country. There are centuries of deep-rooted prejudice to be overcome before the poor people there will listen readily to the truth from our lips ; and, humanly speaking, no agency is better fitted to soften and remove those prejudices, and to open up among them a way for the proclamation of the Gospel message, than the peaceful and benevolent operation of a medical mission.

The next home medical mission was that established in Edinburgh by the late Dr. Handyside, known as "The Main Point Mission Dispensary," the parent of "dear old 39," and, in a sense, of all our home medical mission dispensaries. In a previous chapter, we have related the interesting story of the origin of this medical mission, its removal in 1858 to No. 39, Cowgate, its adoption by the Edinburgh Medical Missionary Society as a Training School for the Society's students, and its subsequent development and success. We proceed now to show the value of this form of agency as an auxiliary to home mission work ; and as facts are better than theories, we may, perhaps, best serve our purpose by giving a few glimpses of our Cowgate work, as carried on from day to day in the " Livingstone Memorial Medical Missionary Training Institution."

Details of equal interest might no doubt be given, regarding the medical missions in London, Glasgow, Birmingham, Bristol, Manchester, and elsewhere. Our object, however, is not so much to give home medical missionary information, as to illustrate the practical working and usefulness of medical missions as a home evangelistic agency, and therefore, in the following pages, we shall confine our attention to the operations of the medical mission in Edinburgh, which it is our privilege to superintend, and with which we are most familiar.

The following summary of cases attended during 1884 will indicate how highly the dispensary is appreciated' and how great a blessing it must be, from a merely benevolent point of view, in the densely populated locality in which it is situated :—

Patients registered only on their first visit  5,477
Patients visited at their own homes    ... 3,243
Midwifery cases attended    ...   ...   ...   236
Vaccination cases  ...         ...   ...   ...   237
                                                    ———
                                    Total  9,193

On the lowest average, each patient came twice to the dispensary for advice at the consulting hour, or to have minor operations performed or wounds dressed at the dispensary hour, thus giving 10,954 visits. The patients treated at their own homes were each visited, at least, three times, thus giving 9,729 separate visits ; adding to this number the attendance on midwifery cases, averaging four visits in each case, upwards of 10,600 visits were paid to the sick at their own homes during the year.

These statistics, which are below the average of several years past, will give some idea of the number of poor people brought, year by year, under the influence of the mission, and imply a vast amount of suffering and misery alleviated or removed; but no statistics can reveal the amount of effort put forth, nor the success of that effort, to lead sin-stricken souls to Jesus, the Great Physician, for spiritual healing. Again and again we have been taught, by the blessed results of faithful, prayerful dealing with our poor patients, that—

> " Down in the human heart,
>     Crushed by the tempter,
> Feelings lie buried that grace can restore ;
>     Touched by a loving hand,
>     Wakened by kindness,
> Chords that were broken will vibrate once more."

Daily, at the consultation hour, may be seen "a great multitude of impotent folk, of blind, halt, withered," waiting their turn, as of old at the pool of Bethesda. The work of each day is begun with a short religious service, conducted by the students, and although the assembly is always a very sad one to behold—poverty, vice, and wretchedness, in all their most aggravated phases, being the prominent feature—yet, as far as regards quiet, respectful attention, and even apparent interest, we could hardly wish a more orderly, or eager audience.

This short service over, the bell rings, and the patients pass, one by one, into the consulting-room, in the order of the number on the ticket which each receives on entering the waiting-room. They are examined, and have suitable medicine prescribed for their ailments, which they receive when they return in the evening. A lady visitor is appointed for each day, who, when the service is over, reads and converses with the patients while any remain in the waiting-room. A few jottings from the pen of one of our lady visitors will give an idea of the interesting and encouraging nature of this labour of love.

"The hours I spend in the waiting-room among the patients I value much, and the work is interesting and varied, reminding one often of the Apostle's words, 'To the one, we are the savour of death unto death, and to the other, the savour of life unto life.' In conversing with them, my first and constant effort is to place before them the Triune Jehovah—a Heavenly Father who cannot look upon sin, but who, while He can only receive the sinner as washed pure in the blood of His dear Son, never fails to remember that we are 'but dust;' a crucified Saviour, now our Advocate with the Father, who is still as willing to plead our cause at God's right hand as when, with His dying breath, He craved forgiveness for those of whom He said, 'they know not what they do;' a Holy Ghost, whose chief delight it is to bring comfort to hearts broken perchance for sin, or by the many

crosses and sorrows of earth.  Sometimes our conversation
will be interrupted by some one saying, 'Oh, the Virgin
will intercede for us!'  Then another of the group of
listeners will say, 'What the lady tells us is quite true;'
or, pointing to a text-card on the wall, another will read
aloud, 'It is a faithful saying, and worthy of all accepta-
tion, that Christ Jesus came into the world to save sinners,'
and others will chime in with, 'Ay, He is the one to
save us.'

"I strive, too, to impress upon their minds the value
and privilege of prayer.  The feelings of two classes
among the patients, on this subject, will best be told as
they were manifested.  On one occasion, the student,
whose turn it was to conduct the usual opening service,
was detained at the infirmary a little beyond two o'clock.
A few minutes after the hour had struck, one woman,
fearing lest the Scripture reading, address, and prayer
should that day be omitted, exclaimed, 'Lady, are we to
have no prayer to-day?'  I instantly felt, that a soul thus
craving to be led into communion with God must have
an effort made to meet its want.  'Yes, my good woman,'
I replied, 'we *shall* have prayer; one of the doctors
always asks a blessing upon *us*—it shall be our privilege
to-day to seek a blessing and wisdom for them.'

"On another occasion, a woman came in just a moment
or two before the student who was to conduct the service
entered.  On learning that, previous to the patients being
called into the consulting-room, there is an address and

17

prayer, she said, ' Oh, I've other things to attend to, I've got no time for prayer.' Catching up her words, I replied, ' No time for prayer! no time for prayer! but one day you will have to find time for death!' She made no reply, but quietly took her seat. After the address, when the student retired, I took advantage of the opportunity, and read some portions of Scripture, and related a few anecdotes illustrating the power of prayer, which seemed to produce a deep impression upon the poor woman, and indeed upon all present.

" I love to place before them the bright prospect, to the child of God, of heaven as a home, for which they must prepare, where there shall be no temptation to sin, where no sorrow shall ever enter, and no pain or sickness shall ever be felt; and as I have thus talked with them, I have seen the big tear trickling down the cheek of one and another, and many times, even strong, rough men have turned (when the bell had rung for them to pass into the consulting-room) to say, ' Good-bye, ma'am, I won't forget what you have been telling us.' Lately, a young woman said to me, ' A friend of mine heard you here the other day talking about these things, and when she came home, she told the whole of it to us.' I could but ask her to go and do likewise. In speaking one day, principally to the children, a mother, pointing to her daughter, said quietly to me, 'She will tell it all over to father to-night, when he comes home from his work.'

" On another occasion, the student read and dwelt upon

the parable of the Prodigal Son; and as I endeavoured
to illustrate it afterwards in a homely way, a man told me
he had known that chapter since he was a child; his
grandfather almost invariably made him read it over to
him on the Sabbath evening; and at school, a well-bound
Bible was offered to the boy who could repeat it most
correctly. He gained the prize, 'and a sixpence besides
from grandfather.' The assurance of pardoned sin—the
realization that we are one with Christ, and He with us—
he could not imagine any one could have; but so en-
grossed was he with the conversation, that when his turn
came, he made ten patients go into the consulting-room
before he went, and at last, when all had been examined
except himself, he begged I would wait till he had seen
the doctor—which I promised to do. On his return to
the waiting-room, he told me he was going to Glasgow
next day. 'We might never meet again on earth,' he
said, 'but, by God's grace, we'll meet in heaven;' and
bidding me good-bye, he promised, if once more back in
Edinburgh, that he would be sure to come to the waiting-
room for more instruction, even should he not need
medicine. Surely within that poor man there was a
thirsting for the truth; may the Weary One who sat on
Jacob's well satisfy him from the river of life."

While visiting patients at their own homes, very
precious opportunities are enjoyed of dealing personally
with many, who might never otherwise care to listen to
the Gospel message; and it is no small pleasure to hear,

from time to time, warm expressions of gratitude from many such, not only for the kind and successful treatment they have received, but likewise for the faithful words spoken to them, and for the prayers offered on their behalf. One or two glimpses of this department of the work may interest the reader.

Within three days, we attended two death-beds, both dispensary cases, and we could not have wished to listen to more satisfactory testimony to the preciousness of Jesus than was given by both these poor patients. In neither case were we present when the spirit took its flight; but the one left a message for us with her husband, who came to the dispensary within half an hour of his wife's death, and faithfully delivered it to us. "Tell the doctor," she said, "that his prayers have been answered, and that Jesus was with me all through the dark valley; tell him I can never, never thank God enough for all the good I have got at the dispensary, for there I came to know my Saviour." The last time she was out was at the Saturday Evening Entertainment, when she got a text, which, she said, was a great source of comfort to her on her dying bed.

The other case was that of a young woman—a great sufferer, but very patient. The day before she died, she tried to express to us how thankful she felt to Dr. B——, who had seen her in consultation several times. "How kind you have both been to me!" she said; "but you have done it all for Jesus, and He says, put it all down to My account. That's a grand text; give it to Dr. B—— from me when you see him next." She alluded to the words, " Inasmuch as ye have done it unto one of the least of these my brethren, ye have done it unto me." Visiting her a few days previously, she said, " No one knows the agony I suffer—it's just like as if you had cut down to the bone of my leg, and then poured in melted lead ; and it never cools, it's burning, burning from night to morning, and from morning till night." We expressed the hope that she would continue to bear her sufferings patiently, when she said, " Oh, doctor, do you think I'm complaining ? I wadna hae it ither than it is for a' the warld. The mair I suffer, the closer I get to Jesus, and it helps me to think of His sufferings for me." She died very peacefully a few days after that interview.

One of our patients who had long been a great sufferer died recently. The day before his death, when we visited him, he said to us : " Doctor, I'm glad to see you once more, and to tell you that I'm perfectly happy, and have no fear. I'm resting on Jesus, the Rock of Ages, and I'll soon be with Him in glory. I want you to tell the students, for their encouragement, that, under God, I owe all to the dispensary, and to the Gospel of His grace which I heard there."

Mrs. K—— was an Irishwoman—one of a class we are daily brought into contact with, and whose surroundings and prejudices are such as to render it almost impossible for the City Missionary or Bible-woman to gain access with the Gospel. The house physician thus writes of her : "I was from time to time called to attend her husband, who is subject to attacks of epileptiform convulsions. I always receive a very kindly welcome from these two, although, on my visits, I invariably have prayer and reading of the Word with them. They listen most attentively, and converse freely about the portions read. The books I lend them are received with gratitude, and perused with care. The old man, whose strength is fast failing, often comes to the door with me to have a few last words, and always entreats me to pray for him ; and now his wife and he attend regularly our meeting on the Sabbath evening.

"Mrs. M—— was a great sufferer, and at first, like Mrs. K——, very strong in her prejudices. By and by, when confidence was established, she allowed me to pray with her. I told her that the Lord Jesus Christ, and only He, was able to save to the uttermost. 'Yes,' she replied with emphasis ; 'only He, only He.' She passed through months of wearying pain, but manifested much patience, receiving, day and night, the kind and gratuitous ministrations of a girl who lodged in the same room with her. Her own daughter—a poor, half-witted creature— could do but little, and her husband was a drunkard. But, ere long, the whole family welcomed us, and the glad tidings we brought to them, and it was most encouraging to see how eagerly even the husband would accept our books and tracts, and begin to read them before our visit was over. Early in the winter she passed away, rejoicing in the assurance that ' He, and He only, can save to the uttermost.'

"Mrs. S—— and her husband belong to the same class, and during the winter they have both been ill, and required frequent visits. They not only listen most attentively to the reading of the Scriptures, but, at their urgent request, I obtained a New Testament for them, and they tell me that they and their son never go to rest at night without reading a portion."

It would be easy to multiply examples of the ready access the medical missionary obtains to a class, otherwise almost inaccessible, in the Cowgate and neighbourhood. These not only gladly welcome him, and receive instruction from him in their homes, but also come to the week-night and Sunday evening services to learn more.

A home medical mission will not be long in operation, before the requirements of the work will necessitate the formation of various schemes of Christian activity and usefulness—all of them intimately associated with, and, indeed, the outcome of, the dispensary practice. These we shall best illustrate by a brief allusion to the different departments of work carried on in connection with the Cowgate Medical Mission.

1. *Evangelistic Services.* Besides the daily service with the patients in the waiting-room, two regular evangelistic

meetings are held weekly, one on Thursday evening, the other on Sunday evening. The attendance fluctuates, but often the Magdalen Chapel is crowded by a very poor, though most attentive audience. An after-meeting is held at the close, and frequently nearly all who are present at the first meeting remain for prayer, and not a few for personal conversation. As the result of these services, many have been awakened, have found peace in believing, and are now proving, by their consistent conduct and enjoyment of Christian privileges, the reality of the change they have experienced.

2. *A Bible Class for Adults* is conducted by one of the senior students on the Sunday afternoon. This class is specially intended for inquirers, and enables us to know those who are really in earnest, so that we can help them, in many ways, amid their numerous difficulties and temptations.

3. *The Sunday Forenoon Children's Church* held in the Magdalen Chapel, and the *Cowgate Arabs' Sunday School* which meets in the waiting-room in the evening, are two of the most hopeful and interesting departments of the work. Every Sunday, between four and five hundred children, living in the Cowgate and neighbour-hood, receive Christian instruction at these services. Many of them, when first laid hold of, are as utterly ignorant of Divine truth as the children in Central Africa, but they have been tamed, and trained, and taught, till now the Cowgate children's services will compare favour-

ably with those held in connection with many of our City churches in more favoured localities. Last year the children attending the Sunday forenoon service contributed no less than £12, to help their former teachers in carrying on their medical mission work in Persia and Kashmir.

The student who superintends the Cowgate Arabs' Sunday Evening School thus writes of its present hopeful condition and prospects: " Implicit and prompt obedience is now secured with comparatively little effort, and if a rebellious spirit should occasionally manifest itself, it is very quickly and effectually quelled, by dealing with the miscreant on the platform in presence of the whole school. Time was, when such a plan of dealing with our unruly boys would have almost inevitably created a riot. An orderly, quiet, and, we believe, profitable service now amply repays us, for the time and labour spent in ' breaking in ' those previously neglected little ones ; and now that we can more and more systematically minister to the needy souls of our youthful charge, we may, humanly speaking, expect that with the Divine blessing fruit will soon appear, and some of the lambs be brought within the fold."

4. *Services in Lodging-Houses.* On Sunday afternoons, meetings are held by the students in several of the large lodging-houses in the Cowgate and Grassmarket. In most of these lodging-houses, patients reside for longer or shorter periods, who during the week are visited, or

come for treatment to the dispensary. Thus we get acquainted with them and their fellow-lodgers, and gaining ready access, we have often in these houses most attentive audiences of from twelve to twenty or thirty people.

5. *The Young Women's Association* is a most encouraging and important department of our work. The management and active work of the association devolve on a president—who is generally the resident physician for the time being—and lady associates, of whom at present there are fourteen. Each lady associate has from eight to ten girls under her special charge, whom she visits regularly. Much good has resulted from the personal influence thus exercised, and many girls have been helped, encouraged, and guided amid the many temptations and difficulties that beset them. One hundred and forty-five members are at present on the roll—as many, indeed, as our limited accommodation will admit of our receiving. The ages of the girls vary from fifteen to twenty-two. The great majority are shop girls, book-folders, and envelope makers ; some are domestic servants, others message girls, while a few who are orphans, or whose mothers are dead, attend to household affairs.

The schemes in operation in connection with the Young Women's Association are Bible classes, a temperance society, missionary sewing-meetings, lectures, a savings' bank, registry for situations, a lending library, and benefit society. A prayer-meeting is held fortnightly, which has been the means of blessing to not a few. Sixty of the girls are members of the "Scripture Union." The weekly meeting of the association is held on Monday evening, in the waiting-room of the institution, when instructive lectures are delivered by members of our medical staff, by returned missionaries, students, or other friends. Examinations are held from time to time on the subjects of lectures, and prizes are awarded. One evening every month is devoted to music, while another, which is greatly enjoyed, is usefully spent as a missionary sewing-meeting. Weekly Bible exercises are regularly written by the members of the Bible class, and two prizes are given, at the close of the summer session, for the best answers to written questions upon the lessons taught during the year. The good influences thus brought to bear upon the young women have been much blessed, and many of them give evidence that they have undergone a saving change.

6. *The Young Men's Association* has only lately been commenced; between thirty and forty young men, from fifteen to twenty-one years of age, have already joined as members, paying a subscription of one penny a week. A reading and recreation room is open three nights a week. Bound volumes of the *Graphic, Good Words, The Leisure Hour, British Workman,* &c., and the daily newspapers, are provided; also a bagatelle table, draught boards, dominoes, &c. Twice a week classes are held

for reading and writing. In this way, we endeavour to offer counter-attractions to those of the public-house, and it is encouraging to find that the members of the association appreciate our efforts in this direction.

7. *Saturday Evening Entertainments* are given regularly once a fortnight during the winter, when the waiting-room is always filled to overflowing, and many of our patients and their friends are thus enabled to close the week, not as it otherwise might be, in rioting and drunkenness, but in a profitable and enjoyable manner. We believe these entertainments have helped to promote the success of the more direct missionary work. We have received letters from several of those who used to attend, but who are now at work in various parts of the country, some of them abroad, telling us that the first step towards a better course of life was taken at these Saturday evening entertainments.

*A Temperance Society* for adults, and a *Band of Hope* for the young, are also important departments of our medical missionary work. No Christian worker among the lapsed masses can do much good, unless he is an out-and-out abstainer, and experience has taught us that the fallen can never be reclaimed, unless by God's grace they are brought to take their stand on the total abstinence platform. Brought as we are into the closest contact with our home heathenism, we would here bear emphatic testimony to the humiliating fact, that amongst the class for whose welfare we labour, the curse of intemperance effectually prevents any general, widespread, permanent impression from being produced upon the community. We worked in the Cowgate, as a student, twenty-five years ago, and although we rejoice to know that since then, by God's blessing on the medical mission and other agencies, not a few have been rescued out of that slough of iniquity, wretchedness, and crime, yet we believe that the Cowgate, with its dismal, dirty closes is no better now, morally and socially, than it was then, and the police statistics of the City confirm this testimony.

Edinburgh, for beauty of situation, for intellectual, moral, and social advantages, for general refinement and high Christian privilege, is second to no city in the kingdom; yet alongside of all this, and in the very heart of this fair metropolis of Scotland, there is a seething mass of wretchedness, pollution, crime, disease, pauperism, and sin, from which, were the veil to be uplifted, and the ghastly spectacle revealed, the exclamation of the prophet of old, concerning guilty Jerusalem, would rise spontaneously to many a lip, "Is this the city that men call the perfection of beauty, the joy of the whole earth?"

In the one short, narrow street in which the medical mission is planted, we have no fewer than twenty-six licensed spirit shops. The poor degraded victims of the "drink crave" cannot resist temptation; their habitual indulgence robs them of self-control, and makes them content to live on in misery and degradation. The mere

sight or smell of alcohol, in the case of those to whom
we refer, is sufficient to create the appetite, and hence,
in a district like the Cowgate, such an array of spirit
shops simply provides unlimited facilities for the complete
demoralization of the community.    Our legislators may
theorize as to the causes of drunkenness, and ascribe the
prevalence of the evil to insanatory dwellings, to neglect
of education, lack of means for healthy recreation, &c.,
but we unhesitatingly affirm, that in the case of those at
least, who have fallen so low as to have become the
denizens of our city slums, the supply creates the demand.
Under existing circumstances, therefore, the moral and
social reformation of such districts is physiologically, as
well as morally, impossible.    In legislative action which
admits, and even fosters, such a state of matters in our
midst, we are not only openly setting at defiance the laws
of Christian morality, but likewise the first principle of
civil government, which, as defined by a great living
statesman, is "to make it easy to do right, and difficult
to do wrong."

Upon the Church of Christ, which should be "fair as
the moon, clear as the sun, and terrible as an army with
banners," there rests a heavy responsibility in regard to
this national sin—the greatest of all obstacles to the
success of home mission work.    Statesmen may legislate,
and social reformers may agitate, for the limitation or
suppression of the drink traffic, and we hail their co-
operation, and bid them God-speed in their zealous

efforts; but our hope rests in the Church of Christ rising to the dignity of her calling, and exerting her mighty influence against this God-dishonouring and soul-destroying sin, which is such a blot upon our national escutcheon.

There is cause for congratulation that the Church of Christ, in its various sections, is becoming more and more alive to the importance of this question, in its relation to home evangelization ; but her testimony must be more clear and emphatic, and her efforts more united and sustained, before this giant evil can be overcome, and the Gospel have free scope among the sunken masses, to bear its own testimony to its all-conquering power.

We have made this digression in order to record our conviction that, with the existing legislation, and the present system of administering the licensing laws, the Church in her aggressive work among the lapsed masses is utterly powerless, so far as that work aims at the reclamation of the moral wastes of our home heathenism. Unless a radical change is effected, so that instead of multiplying temptations they may, as far as possible, be removed from the haunts of the drunken and depraved, the Church should no longer hide from herself the humiliating fact, that while here and there one and another may, by God's blessing, be rescued, yet, so far as her regenerating influence upon such communities is concerned, her efforts are hopeless. We believe that the lamentable want of success in home mission work is mainly owing to the Church's lethargy and indifference in regard to this one great evil. We are reaping as we have sown. God deals with the Church in her collective capacity as he deals with individuals, "He that soweth to his flesh shall of the flesh reap corruption." "If thou forbear to deliver them that are drawn unto death and those that are ready to be slain; if thou sayest, Behold we knew it not; doth not He that pondereth the heart consider it, and He that keepeth thy soul, doth not He know it? and shall not He render to every man according to his works?" (Prov. xxiv. 11, 12.)

Regular weekly meetings are held in connection with the Medical Mission Temperance Society and Band of Hope. The fortnightly Saturday evening entertainments, at which Gospel temperance addresses are alway given, have been the means of bringing many forward to sign the pledge; and opportunities are likewise afforded at the close of the Thursday and Sunday evening evangelistic services. Good has also been done in some instances, by the distribution of attractive temperance literature, such as *The British Workman*, *The Welcome*, "The Life of J. B. Gough," and other periodicals and tracts. Looking back on what has been done in this department of the medical mission work, in the way of reclaiming from drunkenness, and from the depths of misery and wretchedness, those for whom Christ died, we have cause for thankfulness. We have had discouragements not a few, in the falling away of some who, for a time, seemed to be getting on well; but, on the other hand, we have again and again had the great joy of seeing men and women firmly resisting temptation, and, under the influence of Divine Grace, entering, we believe, upon a new and better course of life.

The Band of Hope is carried on with regularity and energy, but while such work among the young is always the most hopeful, yet when we remember the surroundings of these poor children in the Cowgate, can we wonder that their goodness is too often as "a morning cloud, and as the early dew it goeth away?"

While volunteer help from friends outside is always welcome, and indeed in some departments of our work necessary, the various schemes in connection with the Mission Dispensary are worked by small committees of our students appointed at the commencement of each session; and while all are expected, and do heartily co-operate, to secure the success of the work as a whole, yet each committee is responsible only for the regular and efficient working of its own department.

In the Cowgate Medical Mission two objects have to be kept in view. It is not merely a local benevolent and evangelistic agency, but likewise a training school for our future medical missionaries; and in order to afford the students sufficient scope for gaining practical medico-evangelistic experience a variety of work is necessary. During his four years' course of preparation, each student has his share of responsibility and of work in connection with all the schemes in operation. He goes forth to the foreign field, not as a novice, but as a trained and tested medical missionary, having an intelligent grasp of the medical mission principle, and familiar with the best methods of carrying on medico-evangelistic work. It has been our aim to make the Cowgate Medical Mission a model mission dispensary — a mode alike for the home and the foreign field; and the best evidence of its usefulness is the fact, that the Cowgate Mission Dispensary is reproduced, with more or less identity of detail wherever, in this or in other lands, its students are engaged in their Christ-like work.

A home medical mission should begin its work on a small scale, allowing its operations gradually to expand, and each new department to grow out of the other. Funds will be forthcoming, and workers will assuredly offer themselves just as the need may arise. There are many Christian physicians in practice in our larger towns and cities who would be willing, no doubt, to give their professional services at the dispensary an hour or more a day, as is done in Edinburgh; and there are likewise Christian ladies and gentlemen in full sympathy with the poor, who, out of love for their Saviour, would be ready to do all the rest. In its inaugural stages at least, a home medical mission might thus be established, even in our smaller towns, and with very little expense. There is one point to which special importance should be attached, namely, that the mission be conducted on strictly unsectarian principles. Representatives from all the Evangelical churches in the community should form its committee of management, and workers from all denominations should be invited to co-operate in carrying on the work.

Injudicious charity, of whatever kind, is hurtful, and tends to pauperize the recipients and undermine their self-respect. Even in providing medical relief for the poor, this has to be kept in mind, and assuredly a medical mission, if established on the provident system, will prove all the more a beneficent agency. The aid received will be none the less appreciated, while the moral influence of the institution will be greatly increased. While, therefore, a small fixed charge for the medicine dispensed (say twopence or threepence) will tend to foster self-help among the patients, it will also largely help to defray the expense of the drug bill. The patients who seek advice at a mission dispensary belong, no doubt, to the poorest class, but poor, wretched and miserable as they are, they seem never at a loss for the means to supply themselves with whisky, and therefore, when the rule is once adopted, that a small fixed payment is to be made for the medicine, it should be firmly and impartially adhered to, and exceptions made, only in very special circumstances, and after very careful inquiry.

Home medical missionary dispensaries ought to be much more numerous than they are, and should be recognized as an essential department of city mission work.

Through the early and middle ages the Christian Church was the great eleemosynary institution; provision for the poor, the alleviation of physical suffering and distress, medical aid for the destitute sick, all came directly from the Church, and in this ministry, the teaching of the New Testament and the example of Christ were the sources of her inspiration. The Reformation, in its protestation against the doctrine of "Good Works," relegated religion, for the most part, entirely to the heart, and left the relief of the sick and suffering poor to the tender mercies of the State, or impersonally, to the whole body of citizens, and hence the medical relief of the poor has lost its distinctively Christian character. There is no lack of the charitable relief of suffering in connection with our public hospitals and dispensaries, but it is now merely a matter of relief, while its bestowment has little practical value as an influence over human hearts, and is not made to bear with it, as in olden times, the odour of the love of God. Happily, in our mission fields abroad, the Church is reverting to her earlier, more Christ-like method of work, and in so doing she is reaping a rich reward. In many parts of the world, a devoted medical missionary can do more in a month to commend the Gospel, than an ordinary missionary in the same community could do in a year; and experience and observation alike teach that, hand in hand with the Gospel, the healing art will be found of equal value in our mission fields at home.

It is not enough merely to acknowledge that these

institutions—our hospitals, our asylums, and refuges—
are the outcome of Christianity; this, they undoubtedly
are, and, not infrequently, their benevolent operations
are conducted by ministers of the Gospel, by Christian
physicians, and by devoted business men : but the rightful
place, which all such institutions should occupy, is that of
auxiliaries to Christian work, and their blessings should
be dispensed as the direct outcome and manifestation of
the love and sympathy of Christ. Viewed in this light,
medical missions sustain that true relation to human suffering which is, we believe, the Divine intention, and the
practical outcome of the Gospel of the Great Healer.

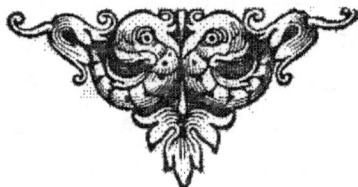

# CONCLUSION.

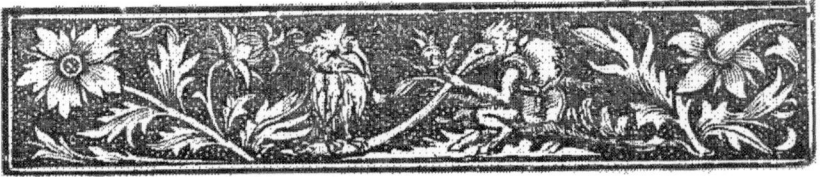

## CHAPTER X.

### Appeal to Young Men, to Students, and to the Friends of Missions.

WE have, in these pages, endeavoured to plead the claims of Medical Missions. We have advocated the more general employment of this agency, on the ground that it is a method of missionary work not only sanctioned, but enjoined, by the Master Himself, and that the compassionate spirit of the Gospel claims, on behalf of the less favoured nations, languishing in misery and superstition, the consecration of medical science and skill. We have illustrated the value of this agency, alike as a pioneer to missionary work, and as a direct means of bringing the truth to bear upon the heart and conscience of individuals; and we have seen that medical missions are no mere experiment, but that they have been tried and tested in almost every land, and among the most prejudiced and exclusive communities, and,

moreover, that they have been most signally owned and
blessed of God, in the furtherance of His cause and
kingdom.    The claims of the missionaries themselves
and their families, no less than our duty to the native
converts in their times of sickness, have been presented
as a powerful plea, for the establishment of a medical
department in connection with every localized mission.
The history and progress of modern medical missions
have been traced, in the establishment and growth of the
Edinburgh Medical Missionary Society, and in the wide-
spread interest in the cause which is now manifested;
and lastly, while our chief object has been to promote
the Foreign Medical Missionary enterprise, we have not
overlooked the claims of medical missions as an auxiliary
to Home Evangelization, while throughout we have endeavoured to set forth the principles which impart to this
agency, whether employed at home or abroad, its peculiar
value and importance.

To take advantage of the openings for the employment
of this agency which, in the providence of God, are
everywhere presented, many more medical missionaries
are required, and to the Christian youth of our country
our appeal must therefore be made.

In this truly benevolent and Christ-like work, an opportunity is presented of consecrating the highest skill,
and the noblest powers, to the service of the best of
Masters, and to the promotion of the holiest and grandest
of enterprises.    "The harvest truly is plenteous, but the

labourers are few; pray ye therefore the Lord of the harvest, that He will send forth labourers into His harvest." Men and women endowed with special gifts and graces are needed. We have elsewhere indicated the difficult and responsible nature of the medical missionary's work, and the peculiar temptations to which he is exposed, it is not therefore necessary again to refer to these. The promise of " grace sufficient" is set over against every difficulty and every temptation, however great or strong, and will enable the faithful follower of the Lord Jesus to say, with the great Apostle : " Most gladly, therefore, will I rather glory in my infirmities, that the power of Christ may rest upon me, for when I am weak, then am I strong."

Our appeal is not addressed to young men who have a high estimate of their own ability, and who make light of the difficulties and responsibilities of the work. Such men, however richly endowed with gifts and graces, make but poor representatives of the Master anywhere, but especially so in the mission field. One of the truest and most reliable evidences of a call from God to engage in this service, is a humble sense of one's own insufficiency, which can only be met with the Divinely inspired conviction, " Our sufficiency is of God."

From every land is wafted the Macedonian cry, " Come over and help us," while with that cry is heard the pitiful wail of languishing humanity. Men are needed, to go forth to those neglected and suffering millions, with

healing in the one hand and the Gospel in the other—
men skilled as physicians, and wise to win souls—men
filled with love to Christ, and with the Spirit of the living
God—men upon whom the spirit of the great Apostle
rests, constraining them to esteem the work as a "grace
given," not as a duty imposed—as a privilege enjoyed,
not as a sacrifice made. Such young men the Church
needs, and to such God, in His providence, now appeals.
"Whom shall I send, and who will go for us? saith the
Lord." Oh that from our universities, our medical schools,
our halls of learning ; from the workshop, the counter,
and the desk, many young men, impelled by the constraining influence of the love of Christ, may respond,
"Here am I, Lord, send me."

To those who are about to enter the profession, and
to young graduates on the outlook for a suitable sphere
in which to commence practice, the Divine call comes,
and we ask such to consider the claims of this department of service. We address ourselves to those who, by
God's grace, reckon themselves "debtors to the Gospel,"
and looking to the "fields white unto the harvest," all
we would ask of such is, to inquire conscientiously and
prayerfully, "Lord, what wilt thou have me to do? Am I
fitted, and if fitted, am I willing, to devote my life to this
service?" Let such questions be pondered calmly and
prayerfully, and we may rest assured that, to such as
are called of God to go forth into the field, the way will
be made plain before them, and they will receive the

special equipment needed for the special work assigned
to them; while those, who are unable to go, will receive
the comforting assurance that, if there be "the willing
mind" it is accepted according to what a man hath, and
not according to what he hath not.

It may touch a chord in the heart of some young
Christian physician, for whom God has yet higher and
nobler service in store than he has ever contemplated;
and it may serve as an inspiration to others, and as an
appeal to their loyalty and devotion to Christ, if we here
relate the experience of Dr. Asahel Grant, to whose remarkable success as a medical missionary, reference has
been made in a previous chapter. In his "Appeal
addressed to Pious Physicians," written soon after his
arrival in Persia, Dr. Grant thus alludes to the time when
he decided to leave all for Christ, and to go forth as a
medical missionary. "A young physician, who had an
extensive and increasing practice in one of our flourishing
cities, had thought much of engaging in the work, but as
often as he considered the matter he dismissed it, under
the plea that, much as labourers might be needed, yet
there were so many obstacles in *his* way, that *he*, at all
events, could not go. Others were better qualified, and
had far less to detain them at home—they might go;
but they did not—the call was urgent, and what was to
be done? He prayed over the subject, and resolved on
a more thorough examination of personal duty. He
took up his former excuses one by one. He asked, can

I do more at home or abroad for the conversion of the world ? In this view, where am I most needed ? Here, I may relieve much suffering, and perhaps prolong some valuable lives ; but should I go, others could do that just as well, and I should not be missed. Abroad, I may relieve a hundred-fold more of misery, perhaps save the lives of missionaries, of inestimable value to the cause, and that, too, when no one else will do it. Here, I have many opportunities of working for Christ, but what are they in comparison with those abroad, where I may be the only spiritual guide to thousands who would never be reached by another. Here, if I prosper, I can give liberally, and labour for the heathen by proxy ; but money alone will not do the work, and labourers, especially physicians, are not to be found. Here, as an officer in an influential church, and in connection with various benevolent societies, I may do much—and many think I ought not to change a certainty for an uncertainty; but do I not know, that those churches that do the most for the heathen, and send forth the most labourers, are the most blessed of God ? Can I not, then, do most for Christ at home, by going in person to those who sit in darkness ?

" But there are other ties, entwined with the tenderest feelings of nature ; and how shall they be severed ? How shall I leave my parents in their declining years ? How say farewell to my sister and brothers ? More than all, how can I leave two darling children alone in this selfish world ? In these questions, so far as mere feeling is concerned, though the heart thrill with agony, it should not turn the Christian from duty. My parents are not dependent upon me, my going may be the greatest blessing to my brothers and sister, and what can I do for my children that would not be done for them if I am gone? The great thing to be done for a child is to fit him for usefulness here, and for the enjoyment of God in heaven. For this, agencies can be provided, and super-added will be a parent's example, turning their attention to the great work he prays they may be qualified to pursue. If God calls me to leave them for IIis sake, He will take care of them. It may be the duty of others to go, but would I let my neighbour die of hunger, because his rich brother ought to feed him rather than I? No more can I let millions perish, because others do not give them the Bread of Life. I cannot, I dare not, go to judgment, till I have done the utmost God enables me to do, to diffuse IIis glory throughout the earth."

The foreign field needs men like Dr. Asahel Grant, who will calmly count the cost, and whose Christianity inspires them with the determination to honour Christ, by seeking to make the world better—men who solemnly consecrate themselves and all they have to God, and who dare not go from IIis altar, and stand convicted before their own consciences, of having loved the world more than God and the souls of their perishing fellow-men—men who can say, as he said : " My heart almost faints within me, when I think of the magnitude of the work, and of my own unfitness for it; but then, when I remember that He gave Himself for me, and has promised to uphold me, then, at His call, and sustained by the blessed assurance, 'I am with you alway,' I stand ready to go, in the face of danger and of death, to any part of the world under the dominion of the prince of darkness, my only wish in regard to a location being to go where I am most needed."

In this service, no great earthly rewards are promised, no alluring prospects of professional distinction, no tempting retiring allowances; but most inviting fields are offered for the exercise of the highest professional accomplishments, the prospect of a life of exceptional usefulness, and, when life's labour is ended, the " Well done, good and faithful servant." There is, besides, the honour and privilege of being called to be a " fellow-worker" with God, an ambassador for Christ, commissioned to be the means, the witness, and the historian of the highest and noblest developments of civilization ! With St. Paul, the medical missionary may well say, "I magnify mine office," for he, of all others, follows most closely in the footsteps of Him of whom it is recorded, " He went about among all the cities and villages, teaching and preaching in their synagogues, and healing all manner of sickness and disease among the people." Contemplate also the grandeur of the medical missionary's aims ; — in the eloquent words of one of the vice-presidents of the Edinburgh Medical Missionary Society, the late Mr.

Miller, Professor of Surgery in the University of Edinburgh, "Think of the brilliant career that opens out before the medical missionary. How noble, by the simple operation for cataract, to 'throw open the darkened windows of the soul, and let the sweet light of heaven into man's otherwise dreary tabernacle !'—but how nobler far, to open the spiritual eye to see the Sun of Righteousness, to behold the Lamb of God ! How kind the art, by vaccination, to deposit in man's earthly frame a particle of wondrous power, whereby a loathsome, and most fatal plague shall be either altogether averted, or rendered mild and tractable when it comes !—but yet how far more kind, to be the means of introducing into the inner man a new and vital principle, more powerful and prophylactic still—the new heart, the Gospel light, the Spirit's grace—whereby the worst of all evils, sin, shall be shorn of its malignant power, shall be subdued and trampled on, routed and driven away ! How blessed is that skill which cures the ulcerous wound, and mitigates the agonies of fell disease !—but how far more blessed, to heal the soul's deadly hurt, and pour the 'balm of Gilead' into the sinner's wounded spirit ! How merciful the hand that safely amputates the unsightly mass of morbid and abnormal growth, whose very weight is burdensome, whose course is deathward !—but what richer mercy far to help, Bunyan-like, to lift that heavier load, which not only oppresses now, but would crush and sink the bearer into endless misery ! How grateful is the

19

task to cure the halting cripple, and make him walk and leap again as if in youth !—but how more glorious far, to recall the wanderer's steps from folly, sin, and death ; to guide his feet into the way of peace ; to show him the old paths, where is the good way, that he may walk therein and find rest for his soul !"

While the practice of the healing art is marked out, in a way more striking than in any former age, as one of the channels through which the blessings of the Gospel are destined to flow forth upon the world, another result of the employment of this agency may be anticipated, which cannot but inspire the enthusiastic Christian practitioner with an ardent desire to engage in the work. The medical missionary's object is two-fold—to preach the Gospel, and to heal the sick ; and while his skill and success as a practitioner are to be made subservient to his evangelistic work, still, his ministry of healing is, in itself, a service which, in the mission field, is of inestimable value. He carries with him, into less favoured and often barbarous lands, the blessings of our great modern improvements in medical and surgical science, and there, he may even be the means of founding schools of medicine which, at no distant day, may be centres of enlightenment and civilization, radiating the benefits of Western science and beneficence throughout the "dark places of the earth." Where medical missions are established, the training of native agents usually forms an important part of the work. In Agra, a Medical Missionary Training Institution is in operation. In the great empire of China, almost the only means by which the Chinese can obtain a medical education, is in connection with our medical missions; while in Syria and Central Turkey, flourishing medical colleges have been established by American missionary societies. In Japan, while all native physicians, at present practising in the country, may continue to do so according to the system in which they have been trained, a recent order of the Government enforces, that no licenses to practise are in future to be granted except to those who shall pass an examination in Western medical science. There are, according to the official census, thirty-four thousand native physicians practising in Japan, of whom less than five hundred have received any instruction in European medical science. If, therefore, Japan is to be supplied with educated physicians in a proportion equal to its population, before the close of the next generation at least thirty thousand men must be trained, who, from the nature of their profession, will exercise a vast influence upon society. Japan is calling for the medical science of Christendom, and doubtless the call will be responded to, but shall it be with, or without, the faith of Christendom? With God's blessing, a Christian medical school in Japan, such as the Protestant college at Beyrout, and at Aintab in Central Turkey, would prove a most powerful agency in the evangelization of that great empire. The coming era of the missionary enterprise will, we believe, be char-

acterized by a concentration of effort in the great
work of training native agents for the evangelization of
their fellow-countrymen; and in this special department
of work, as in all others, the friends of missions must be
prepared to provide native Christians with the means of
education and training in order to fit them for efficient
service. What inviting spheres of influence and usefulness are thus waiting to be occupied by young talented
medical men, competent to instruct others in their profession, and inspired with the true missionary spirit!
There is scarcely any limit to the hopes that may be
cherished, if, with the Divine blessing, advantage be
taken of the openings in the foreign field for the exercise
of the evangelistic and benevolent operations of the
medical missionary. Surely a work so full of promise,
and so practical, so suited to the requirements of the
mission field, so Apostolic, so Christ-like, claims the
consecration of the noblest powers which our universities
and medical schools can furnish! And to the young man
who may read these pages, especially if he be a medical
student or graduate, we would say, "Think of this work,
dwell upon its glorious issues, look at its claims in the
light of what you owe to Christ, and if you hear the voice
of God calling you to engage in it, manfully take up your
cross, and go forth to it, and you will never cease to
thank Christ Jesus our Lord for counting you worthy to
take part in this ministry."

There has been, of late, an increased and growing in-

terest in the cause of missions, among the educated youth
of our country, the outcome of a wonderful work of Divine
grace among the students of our Universities. This work
is so manifestly of God, that we shrink from referring to
any mere human agency in connection with it; but there
can be no doubt that, while other influences were at work
preparing the way, the blessing came through the channel
of consecrated missionary zeal, on the part of the little
band of devoted men from Oxford and Cambridge Universities, who, constrained by the love of Christ, forsook
all, to live and labour, and, if need be, to die for Him, in
the high places of the field. A work thus inaugurated,
and thus owned of God, cannot but be fraught with rich
blessings to the cause of missions. In view of this missionary revival among students, and of the world's needs,
there rests upon the Church of Christ, and upon our
missionary societies, a great responsibility. At no former
period, have there been so many thoughtful, earnest, and
devoted young men offering themselves for foreign missionary service. Among medical students especially, this
spirit of self-consecration is manifested in a very remarkable degree. The Church has long been praying the
Lord of the harvest "to send forth more labourers into
His harvest;" and now, in the widespread interest in the
cause of missions awakened in our colleges, God is
answering her prayers, and inclining the hearts of many
accomplished and devoted young men to respond to the
Divine call. Is the Church prepared to receive such an

answer to her prayers? Are these young candidates for
missionary service to be encouraged to come forward in
ever-increasing numbers? Is the Church ready to
welcome them, to train them for her service, and to
send them forth as her messengers to the heathen? All
this, of course, implies the provision of vastly increased
resources, and we leave these questions to be pondered,
and prayed over by the friends of missions.

In this blessed work among students, God is teaching
His people, that the way to secure a revival of true godli-
ness in the Church is to cherish the spirit of self-consecration, and to yield a loyal obedience to the Divine
command, " Go ye into all the world, and preach the
Gospel to every creature." The more the heart responds
to the call of humanity, and of Christ, the more room
will be found in that heart for the Divine blessing ; and
the more the Church exerts herself for the extension of
Christ's kingdom abroad, the more will the Holy Spirit's
influence be felt within the Church at home, operating
for her advancement and prosperity. Let the Church
rise to the dignity of her calling, and gathering up all her
mighty resources, seize the present opportunity ; then,
assuredly, "times of refreshing" will come from the
presence of the Lord ; the Lord will give the word, and
"great shall be the company of them that publish it."
" God shall bless us, and all the ends of the earth shall
fear Him."

This plea on behalf of medical missions cannot more

appropriately be concluded, than in the eloquent words of one to whom the cause was very dear, and whose once familiar voice was often heard, advocating the consecration of medical science and skill to the advancement of the Redeemer's kingdom. Speaking at one of the annual meetings of the Edinburgh Medical Missionary Society, Professor Miller said :—

" When we come before you with Scripture warrant on our side—with the personal example of our Lord and His Apostles not only beckoning us on, but reproving us for not having come—with the successful experience of medical missions, as far as they have yet been tried, speaking strongly in our favour, and with the united and cordial approval of every missionary with whom we have ever come in contact—when missionaries all tell us that they find the medical element so essential to the success of their work, that they are compelled sometimes to practise it themselves—when labourers from all quarters of the missionary field, men gallantly bearing the burden and heat of the day, are calling to us anxiously for medical colleagues, not on account of their own health, but to assist them in their great work of reaching the hearts of men whose souls they seek to save—when, had we but the means and the men, we might now plant, not one, or two, or three, but many medical missions in the very heart and strongholds of heathenism, and they would be gladly welcomed, and by and by supported, by the very heathen themselves—with such claims as these, surely it is neither unbecoming nor unwarrantable that we ask earnestly and importunately for your sympathy and aid. And bear with me, if I remind you that you have an important duty to discharge towards the medical profession, that you owe it a debt. Is there any one here who does not feel and acknowledge that debt? Has no father, or brother, or sister, or husband, or wife, or child, been saved to you, under God's providence, by the skill and care of the physician? At a time when all seemed dark and hopeless, and you dared not look into the future, at a time when the blackness of despair had settled down, and wellnigh shut out heaven from your sight, and prayer from your lips, at a time when you would gladly have given all the earthly treasure you possessed, or ever might possess, in barter for the life which seemed so fast and hopelessly ebbing away, has not the physician then seemed to you as a ministering angel sent to comfort you? have you not then clung to him as your best earthly friend, your only earthly hope and stay? And when success attended his efforts in battling with disease and death, and life, and hope, and health came smiling back, have you not wet his hand with your tears of gratitude, and sent him away laden with your blessing and your prayers? Or was it your own life that was quivering in the balance at a time, perhaps, that a downward turn would have hazarded a double death; but when the upward cast, still due apparently to the hand of the physician, bade you live again for time and for eternity? Ah, then, surely the argument we now venture to use, will come home with a double force. Each one who has felt this, or aught like this, will surely acknowledge a large and growing debt of obligation. Let those debts be all accumulated into one vast whole—not due, or at least not to be rendered, to the individual man, but to the God-like profession which they represent. The opportunity is given you to discharge in some measure that debt now. Honours, in old times, were freely accorded to individual practitioners of renown; medals were struck in their honour, bearing the legend '*ob cives servatos*' on account of citizens preserved. We seek no such personal gifts, but we ask you to honour the profession, by helping it to honour and adorn itself, by helping it to write on the bells of the horses 'Holiness unto the Lord,' by helping it to be instrumental in saving the souls as well as the bodies of men, by helping it to place in its coronet new jewels of greatest value and of brightest lustre, by helping it to twine in its garland a new wreath from the ever-green and ever-growing Plant of Renown. And let me add that, in thus honouring the profession, you will honour also that profession's Head. Medicine has been at no time without her gods. The early Greeks owned Apollo; after him came Æsculapius; and gods and demigods followed in abundance. But the power of advancing civilization struck away those unsightly capitols from the otherwise goodly column; not to leave it mutilated and bare, but to make way for the true headstone, to exalt and acknowledge the Great Physician, Jehovah-Rophi, the Lord the Healer—no mythical personage, but He who in very deed dwelt with men upon the earth, who 'went about continually doing good,' and who has promised to be with His faithful followers 'alway, even unto the end of the world.' Such is the double debt and double duty which we ask you now in part, at least, to discharge. But do not mistake the nature of the claim which we make. We seek your pecuniary aid to carry on this great and noble enterprise so beneficent to men, so glorifying to God; but we do not want your money only. 'Your money or your life' is the startling demand of the highwayman; ours is more startling still, 'Your money *and* your life.' Of some select, gifted, and gallant few, we seek their lives wholly devoted, to the death if need be, in the service of their great Master. But of all, we seek their life in one sense, in the sense of claiming that on which true life depends, that whereby spiritual life is fed and maintained, without which it dies—prayer, intercession at the Throne of Grace! . . . And if it be true, that the deadly conflict is now at hand between truth and error, between the powers of light and the powers of darkness, if the time is now near, when we shall be involved as combatants for very life in that eventful struggle, how can we look for Heaven's aid, how dare we ask it, unless we be on Heaven's side, and doing the will of Him who sits Almighty there? How can we in the shock of the coming battle, and in the turmoil of the approaching fray, be otherwise than helpless and overborne, unless, as faithful soldiers of the cross, we be found mustered around, and fighting under, the banner of the Captain of the hosts of the Lord, following where that banner leads, losing neither sight nor hold of it—the banner of Him, whose latest command it was, whose very watchword of the fight is, 'Go ye into all the world, and preach the Gospel to every creature.'

" And He sent them to preach the Kingdom of God, and to heal the sick. . . . And they departed, and went through the towns, preaching the Gospel and healing everywhere " (Luke ix. 2–6).

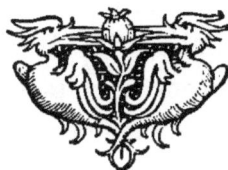

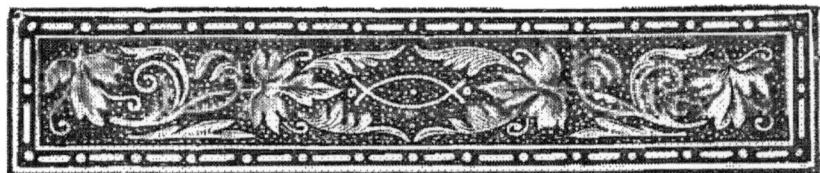

# INDEX.

UNWIN BROTHERS, GRESHAM PRESS, CHILWORTH AND LONDON.

www.ingramcontent.com/pod-product-compliance
Lightning Source LLC
Chambersburg PA
CBHW021508210326
41599CB00012B/1172